MEDITERRANEAN
DIET

*Mediterranean Diet Recipes,
Mediterranean Diet Cookbook and
Mediterranean Diet for Beginners*

7 DAY MEDITERRANEAN DIET MEAL PLAN INCLUDED!

VALERIE CHILDS

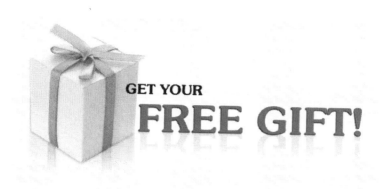

GET YOUR
FREE GIFT!

WAIT! – DO YOU LIKE FREE BOOKS?

My **FREE Gift** to You!! As a way to say **Thank You** for downloading my book, I'd like to offer you more **FREE BOOKS!** Each time we release a NEW book, we offer it first to a small number of people as a test - drive. Because of your commitment here in downloading my book, I'd love for you to be a part of this group. You can join easily here ➔ http://rapidslimdown.com/

Table of Contents

What is the Mediterranean Diet?

The Mediterranean Diet focuses on the Southern countries of Europe (Greece, Turkey, Italy ect) and the emphasis these countries place on high vegetable and fish intake and low meat intake. These countries report the lowest heart disease reports globally. This diet that is rich in healthy fats and produce is also a great way to lose weight and manage weight.

If improving your heart health and lower your risk for diabetes isn't enough, people following a Mediterranean diet also have an increase in energy.

If you choose to follow the Mediterranean diet, you will see improved results in your overall health. You MUST stick with the plan to see the results. A healthy diet and some general activity will go a long way. Now let's get to the GOOD stuff! Here is a small sampling of a 7-day meal plan. The book has wonderful recipes and tips for keeping on track and making this plan simple and easy to follow.

The Mediterranean diet has historically been associated with good health. The food patterns that were typical of Greece resulted in life expectancy that ranked as the highest in the world. In addition, the instances of coronary artery disease and certain cancers were among the lowest in the world. If that wasn't enough praise for this way of eating, the rates of obesity were also extremely low due to a healthy, active lifestyle of an older population. Everyone wondered what they ate and how they were able to stay so healthy and so fit into their later years.

The Mediterranean Diet was characterized by a great many plant foods. The fresh fruits and vegetables were accompanied by oils, nuts, fresh, unprocessed dairy products, fish and poultry, and wine. A diet low in saturated fats, the Mediterranean Diet became famous for its palatability—offering recipes of extraordinary taste.

While variations of this diet exist throughout the regions of Italy, Spain, Syria, Portugal, and Turkey, the diet specifically in Crete was closely tied to the olive production, seasonally grown foods, and unprocessed meats and dairy products that were organically grown and cultivated.

Studies showed that this diet, when consumed in the proper amounts, provided every essential element of nutrition believed to promote health. Moreover, studies found that the foods that were eaten in the Mediterranean Diet were so numerous, with nutrition so complex, that the interaction and synergistic effects of them were too complex to be fully understood. With olive oil as the principal source of fat, it offered the antioxidant vitamin E, enhancing taste and energy density.

Dairy products were typically eaten in low to moderate amounts in Crete. Milk was not available so readily as it is here due to problems of heat and refrigeration, and typically the fresh milk from goats was eaten as yogurts and cheese, grated lightly over pastas rather than eaten in large quantities.

Meat was often scarce, and though it was included in the Mediterranean diet, red meat was taken in low amounts. More often, seafood and fish was on the daily menu. Studies on the diet and the population of Crete actually found that though they ate red meat, the fruits and vegetables that they also included had an antioxidant effect, allowing the inclusion of that protein without adverse effects. Moderate wine consumption and long, lingering meals among family and friends were the final areas studied in the Mediterranean diet. All of these elements together produced a healthful dietary tradition that has become a source of study and a way of living that others have struggled to replicate.

Why choose the Mediterranean Diet?

Research shows that American health is on the decline. Research from CDC.com shows:

- About 610,000 people die of heart disease in the United States every year–that's 1 in every 4 deaths.

- Heart disease is the leading cause of death for both men and women. More than half of the deaths due to heart disease in 2009 were in men.1

- Coronary heart disease is the most common type of heart disease, killing over 370,000 people annually.

- Every year about 735,000 Americans have a heart attack. Of these, 525,000 are a first heart attack and 210,000 happen in people who have already had a heart attack.

- Diabetes is also on the rise in America. We have a fast food, deep-fried addicted to sugar and soda complex and it's showing on our waistlines, and on our health overall.

- The Mediterranean Diet has been shown again and again to correlate directly to the reduced risk of stroke. Studies have theorized that the inclusion of olive oil in the diet may be responsible for this statistic. In fact, the population of Greece and the surrounding areas eat almost no butter, with olive oil providing the primary source of fat in the diets.

Countries such as Greece, Turkey, and Italy, the countries based on the Mediterranean diet, reported the lowest heart disease rate globally. Foods with healthy fats, rich in produce and whole grains help keep metabolisms up and also protect the heart and brain. Learning the basics of a Mediterranean diet will help ensure success in sticking with this proven, healthy diet.

What are the benefits of the Mediterranean Diet?

The Harvard Health blog looked at the benefits of the Mediterranean Diet. Researchers looked at the dietary habits of more than 10,000 women in their 50s and 60s and compared them to how the women fared health-wise 15 years later. Women who followed a healthy diet during middle age were about 40% more likely to live past the age of 70 without chronic illness and without physical or mental problems than those with less-healthy diets. The healthiest women were those who ate more plant foods, whole grains, and fish; ate less red and processed meats; and had limited alcohol intake. That's typical of a Mediterranean-type diet, which is also rich in olive oil and nuts. The report appeared yesterday in the *Annals of Internal Medicine*.

Why would your menu in middle age protect your health later in life? "Several mechanisms may be involved, including lowering inflammation and oxidative stress, both systemically and within the central nervous system. These are two general pathways underlying many age-related chronic diseases and health conditions, such as age-related brain diseases and mental health. Other potential mechanisms include notably improving glucose metabolism and insulin sensitivity," explains lead author Cécilia Samieri, a researcher at Université Bordeaux in France, who conducted the study while a postdoctoral fellow at Harvard Medical School.

Good food is a pretty powerful health booster. Whole grains, legumes, fruit, and vegetables are packed with fiber, which slows digestion and helps control blood sugar. Monounsaturated fats in olive oil, nuts, and fish can have anti-inflammatory effects, which may help stave off heart disease and many other conditions.

Studies show that a high degree of adherence to a strictly Mediterranean diet may decrease mortality and eliminate disease. Each of these components on their own was not enough. For example, you can't simply drink more red wine and expect to lose weight and live longer. However, together they affect a powerful combination that research has shown to have amazing biological benefits. Moreover, the effects are even greater among older age groups than they are among the younger.

Key Points

Key points of the Mediterranean diet plan include:

- Fruits and vegetables: Make the backbone of every meal.

- Whole grains: Use to round out a plate at mealtime.

- Spices: Add for flavor and nutrients with every meal.

- Beans: Include as a daily staple.

- Nuts: Eat a handful as a snack or in a meal every day.

- Olive and canola oil: Use instead of butter and margarine.

- Dairy products: Eat in moderation.

- Red wine: Enjoy one glass with supper or dinner.

Snacks, chips, and dips are not part of this diet plan.

Meal Tips

Here are some tips to help you include choices from the Mediterranean diet when you plan your meals:

Choose fruits and vegetables, at least 6 to 7 servings each day. (Aim for 2-1/2 cups of vegetables and 2 cups of fruit daily.) Look for brightly colored produce that is in season.

- Eat 1 to 2 servings of green leafy vegetables — such as kale, spinach, and leafy salad greens — each day. Green leafy vegetables are full of antioxidants, vitamin C, and folic acid.

- Include some type of fresh salad with most meals.

- Use tomatoes in salads and flavorful sauces.

- Have a 6-ounce glass of citrus fruit juice or vegetable juice every day.

- Use Romaine or spinach as a base for salads.

- Limit potatoes to one serving a week.

- Choose fruit for dessert. Buy fresh melons, berries, oranges, apples, pears, plums, apricots, peaches, papaya, and mangos when they're in season. Many of these are also great frozen.

Starting the Mediterranean Diet

Staples of the Mediterranean Diet

Quinoa

Red onion

- Lemons

- Kalamata olives

- Cucumber

- Cherry Tomatoes

- Feta

- Chicken

- Tomatoes

- Basil leaves

- Penne pasta- whole-wheat

- Garlic

- Brown lentils

- Thyme

- Parsley

- Bacon

- Pine Nuts

- Halibut

- Chicken stock

- Carrots

Eggs

Zucchini

Walnuts

Almonds

Bell peppers

Whole-wheat pita bread

Garbanzo beans

Olive oil

Artichoke hearts

Oats

Bananas

Honey or agave

Apples

Greek Yogurt

Flax seeds

Whole-wheat flour

Shrimp

Chickpeas

Lemons

Eggplants

Olives

Mozzarella cheese

These are staples. Check the recipes you select each week to make sure have all your ingredients and shop on Saturday. Prep and cook Sunday. You will have healthy meals all week. Enjoy leftover or freeze. If you have a sweet tooth, check out the options for desserts for a snack or after dinner. There are also many side dishes you can choose to add to your main dish available in the book. There are simple tasks you can do to prep for the week easier.

*Make a batch of garbanzo beans to last a week. Or buy canned and rinse well.

*You can also buy minced garlic saving time.

*Cut carrot sticks to last a few days

*Grill chicken/fish/shrimp to last a few days to use in recipes found here

*Prepare enough hummus to have a few days worth on hand. It's a quick, healthy snack and a great spread if you make a grilled chicken pita, or want to eat some vegetables.

*Prepare a soup on Sunday you can eat continually throughout the week for lunches or a dinner (or prep and freeze any leftovers to use in upcoming weeks).

Goal setting

Getting your mind straight: Set goals and always keep the end in mind.

Take a before picture.

Get a small notebook and write down how you are feeling at the moment (tired, worn out etc.)

Have a goal in mind (want to wear that little black dress? Pull it out and hang it in plain view where you will see it everyday

Visually seeing yourself as wearing that dress, or your favorite jeans will help you stay on track. When you feel and look energetic the momentum will keep you going.

Focus on what you CAN eat! Find alternatives for your favorite items. Have a sweet tooth? Enjoy your favorite fruits! Or warm whole-wheat pita bread with some honey or agave to dip! Replace unhealthy oils with heart-healthy olive oil. There are healthier alternatives for everything!

The 7-Day Meal Plan Outline

When following the Mediterranean Diet, here is a week long meal plan. Eating smaller meals every few hours helps the metabolism. Eating the correct foods will help in health heart and weight management. An example day may include:

BREAKFAST

Mediterranean Egg Scramble

Prep time: 15 minutes

Cook time: 25 minutes

Yield: 4 servings

Ingredients:

1 teaspoon olive oil

1 teaspoon butter

3 medium-sized new potatoes, thinly sliced

1/4 large red bell pepper, small diced

8 black olives, chopped

1/4 cup fresh parsley, chopped

1/4 cup fresh ricotta cheese

6 eggs

Salt and pepper to taste

4 slices crusty bread

4 teaspoons butter or extra-virgin olive oil

Instructions:

- In a large nonstick skillet, heat the olive oil and butter to medium-high heat. Add the sliced potatoes and sauté for about 15 minutes or until golden. Add the bell pepper and olives and cook for 4 minutes.

- In a medium bowl, whisk together the parsley, ricotta, and eggs. Pour the egg mixture over the potato mixture, stirring every 30 seconds until firm and set but not dry, about 3 minutes. Salt and pepper the egg scramble to taste.

SNACK

Carrot Sticks & Hummus

Ingredients

Original recipe makes 4 servings

- 1 (15 ounce) can garbanzo beans, drained, liquid reserved

- 1 tablespoon lemon juice

- 1 tablespoon olive oil

- 1 clove garlic, crushed

- 1/2 teaspoon ground cumin

- 1/2 teaspoon salt

- 2 drops sesame oil, or to taste

Blend garbanzo beans, lemon juice, olive oil, garlic, cumin, salt, and sesame oil in a food processor; stream reserved bean liquid into the mixture as it blends until desired consistency is achieved.

LUNCH

Minestrone

Prep time: 15 minutes

Cook time: 6–8 hours

Yield: 8 servings

Ingredients:

1 onion, diced

3 carrots, washed, quartered and sliced into 1/2-inch slices

3 celery stalks, quartered and sliced into 1/2-inch slices

Two 14.5-ounce cans navy beans, drained and rinsed

One 28-ounce can diced tomatoes

4 cups low-sodium chicken stock

4 Italian chicken sausage links, quartered and sliced into 1/2-inch slices

2 sprigs thyme, or 1/2 teaspoon dried thyme

2 bay leaves

1/2 teaspoon dried sage

1 cup orzo or other small pasta

3 zucchinis, quartered and sliced into 1/2-inch slices

1/2 cup freshly grated Parmesan for serving

Salt to taste (optional)

- **Instructions:**

- Stir the onions, carrots, celery, beans, tomatoes, stock, sausage, thyme, bay leaves, and sage together in a 4- to 5-quart slow cooker.

- Cook on low for 6 to 8 hours. During the last 30 minutes of cooking, add the orzo and zucchini and cook for 30 minutes on high or until you're ready to serve. Add salt to taste (if desired).

- Divide the soup among eight bowls, removing the bay leaves. Top each bowl with 1 tablespoon of the grated Parmesan and serve.

Per serving: Calories 382 (From Fat 98); Fat 11g (Saturated 4g); Cholesterol 25mg; Sodium 1178mg; Carbohydrate 50g (Dietary Fiber 10g); Protein 23g.

SNACK

½ cup of nuts (your choice– raw walnuts or raw almonds are the heart-healthiest option)

DINNER

Mediterranean Chicken Wrap

- *Prep Time 10 minutes*

- *Total Time 10 minutes*

- *Yield Serves 1*

Chicken provides a great source of protein, while the tapenade adds healthy fats. Artichoke hearts and tomato bring fiber to the table. The whole-wheat wrap offers a better carb choice than a white wrap.

- **Ingredients:**

- 1 chicken cutlet (3 ounces)

- Coarse salt and ground pepper

- 1 whole-wheat wrap, 10 inches

- 1 tablespoon olive tapenade

- 2 cans artichoke hearts, squeezed dry and thinly sliced

1/2 small tomato, thinly sliced

- 1/4 cup mixed baby greens

Instructions:

Heat broiler with rack 4 inches from heat. Season chicken with salt and pepper and broil until opaque throughout, 4 to 5 minutes; let cool.

Spread bottom of wrap with the olive tapenade. Layer with chicken, artichoke hearts, tomato, and baby greens; season with salt and pepper. Fold tortilla to seal.

If you have your chicken already grilled from Sunday this is a quick and easy dinner to put together.

BREAKFAST

Banana Nut Oatmeal

Ingredients:

¼ cup quick cooking oats

½ cup skim milk

1 teaspoon flax seeds

2 tablespoons chopped walnuts

3 tablespoons honey

1 banana, peeled

Instructions:

You can use walnuts or almonds to top off a bowl of oatmeal in this oatmeal.

Combine the oats, milk, flax seeds, walnuts, honey, and banana in a microwave-safe bowl. Cook in microwave on High for 2 minutes. Mash the banana with a fork and stir into the mixture. Serve hot.

SNACK

½ cup of Greek yogurt

LUNCH

Mediterranean Pasta with Artichokes and Olives

Prep Time 15 minutes

Total Time 25 minutes

Yield Serves 4

Ingredients:

- Coarse salt and ground pepper

- 12 ounces whole-wheat spaghetti

- 2 tablespoons olive oil

- 1/2 medium onion, thinly sliced, lengthwise

- 2 garlic cloves, thinly sliced crosswise

- 1/2 cup dry white wine

- 1 can artichoke hearts, drained, rinsed, and quartered lengthwise

- 1/3 cup pitted kalamata olives, quartered lengthwise

- 1 pint cherry or grape tomatoes, halved lengthwise

- 1/4 cup grated Parmesan cheese, plus more serving

- 1/2 cup fresh basil leaves, torn

Instructions:

Whole-wheat pasta has almost twice the amount of fiber of traditional semolina pasta.In a large pot of boiling salted water, cook pasta until al dente according to package directions. Drain, reserving 1 cup of pasta water. Return pasta to pot.

- Meanwhile, in a large skillet, heat 1 tablespoon oil over medium-high. Add onion and garlic, season with salt and pepper, cook, stirring occasionally until browned, 3 to 4 minutes. Add wine and cook until evaporated, about 2 minutes.

Stir in artichokes and cook until starting to brown, 2 to 3 minutes. Add olives and half of the tomatoes; cook until tomatoes start to break down, 1 to 2 minutes. Add pasta to skillet. Stir in remaining tomatoes, oil, cheese, and basil. Thin with reserved pasta water if necessary to coat the spaghetti. Serve with additional cheese.

SNACK

a piece of fruit (apple)

DINNER

Vegetable and Garlic Calzone

Ingredients:

- 3 asparagus stalks, cut into 1-inch pieces

- 1/2 cup chopped spinach

- 1/2 cup chopped broccoli

- 1/2 cup sliced mushrooms

- 2 tablespoons garlic, minced

- 2 teaspoons olive oil

- 1/2 pound frozen whole-wheat bread dough loaf, thawed

- 1 medium tomato, sliced

- 1/2 cup mozzarella cheese, shredded

- 2/3 cup pizza sauce

Instructions:

Preheat the oven to 400 F. Lightly coat a baking sheet with cooking spray.

In a medium bowl, add the asparagus, spinach, broccoli, mushrooms and garlic. Drizzle 1 teaspoon of the olive oil over the vegetables and toss to mix well.

Heat a large, nonstick frying pan over medium-high heat. Add the vegetables and sauté for 4 to 5 minutes, stirring frequently. Remove from heat and set aside to cool.

On a floured surface, cut the bread dough in half. Press each half into a circle. Using a rolling pin, roll the dough into an oval. On half of the oval, add 1/2 of the sautéed vegetables, 1/2 of the tomato slices and 1/4 cup cheese. Wet your finger and rub the edge of the dough that has the filling on it. Fold the dough over the filling, pressing the edges together. Roll the edges and then press them down with a fork. Place the calzone on the prepared baking sheet. Repeat to make the other calzone.

Brush the calzones with the remaining 1 teaspoon olive oil. Bake until golden brown, about 20 minutes.

Heat the pizza sauce in the microwave or on the stove top. Place each calzone on a plate. Serve with 1/3 cup pizza sauce on the side or pour the sauce over the calzones.

Nutritional analysis per serving

Serving size: 1 calzone

Calories: 270

BREAKFAST

Pancakes

Get a side of whole grains with your Greek yogurt by making a stack of pancakes using the recipe from Oikos. Top them off with fresh fruit, toasted nuts, more Greek yogurt, or sweeten the stack with a dash of syrup. It makes about 6 servings.

Ingredients:

1 cup old-fashioned oats

½ cup all purpose whole wheat flour

2 tablespoons flax seeds

1 teaspoon baking soda

¼ teaspoon salt

2 cups Greek yogurt (plain or vanilla)

2 large eggs

2 tablespoons agave or honey

2 tablespoons canola oil

Syrup, fresh fruit, or other toppings

Instructions:

Combine first five ingredients in a blender and pulse process 30 seconds. Add yogurt, eggs, oil, and agave and blend until smooth.

Let batter stand to thicken, about 20 minutes. (Batter can be prepared up to 1 day in advance; cover batter and refrigerate.)

Heat large non-stick skillet over medium heat. Brush skillet with oil. Working in batches, ladle batter by ¼ cupful into skillet. Cook pancakes until bottoms are golden brown and bubbles form on top, about 2 minutes. Turn pancakes over; cook until bottoms are golden brown, about 2 minutes. Transfer to baking sheet. Keep warm in oven. Repeat with remaining batter, brushing skillet with more butter as necessary. Serve with desired toppings.

SNACK

pear or apple

LUNCH

Mediterranean Shrimp and Pasta

Ingredients:

2 teaspoons olive oil

- Cooking spray

- 2 garlic cloves, minced

- 1 pound medium shrimp, peeled and deveined

- 2 cups chopped plum tomato

- 1/4 cup thinly sliced fresh basil

- 1/3 cup chopped pitted kalamata olives

- 2 tablespoons capers, drained

- 1/4 teaspoon freshly ground black pepper

- 4 cups hot cooked angel hair pasta (about 8 ounces uncooked pasta)

- 1/4 cup (2 ounces) crumbled feta cheese

Instructions:

Heat olive oil in a large nonstick skillet coated with cooking spray over medium-high heat. Add garlic; sauté 30 seconds. Add shrimp, sauté 1 minute. Add tomato and basil; reduce heat, and simmer 3 minutes or until tomato is tender. Stir in kalamata olives, capers, and black pepper.

Combine shrimp mixture and pasta in a large bowl; toss well. Top with cheese.

Nutritional Information

Calories per serving: 424

SNACK

1 cup of pistachios or other nuts

DINNER

Mediterranean Chickpea Patties

Ingredients:

- 1 (15.5-ounce) can chickpeas, rinsed and drained

- 1/2 cup fresh flat-leaf parsley

- 1 garlic clove, chopped

- 1/4 teaspoon ground cumin

- 1/2 teaspoon kosher salt, divided

- 1/2 teaspoon black pepper, divided

- 1 egg, whisked

- 4 tablespoons all-purpose flour, divided

- 2 tablespoons olive oil

- 1/2 cup low-fat Greek-style yogurt

- 3 tablespoons fresh lemon juice

- 8 cups mixed salad greens

- 1 cup grape tomatoes, halved

1/2 small red onion, thinly sliced

Pita chips (optional)

Instructions:

Pulse first 4 ingredients (through cumin) and 1/4 teaspoon each salt and pepper in a food processor until coarsely chopped and mixture comes together. Transfer to a bowl, add egg and 2 tablespoons flour; form into 8 (1/2-inch-thick) patties. Place remaining flour in a small dish and roll patties in it with floured hands; tap off excess flour.

Heat oil in a nonstick skillet over medium-high heat. Cook patties for 2-3 minutes per side or until golden.

Whisk together the yogurt, lemon juice, and remaining salt and pepper. Divide greens, tomatoes, onion, and patties evenly among 4 plates; drizzle each salad with 2 tablespoons dressing. Serve with pita chips, if desired.

Calories per serving:	225
Fat per serving:	8g

BREAKFAST

Chickpea and Potato Hash

This hash will be a suitable meal choice anytime of the day, including breakfast. It will certainly keep you full, containing 14 grams of protein, and 6 grams of fiber per serving; it will make enough for 4 people.

Ingredients:

4 cups frozen shredded hash brown potatoes

2 cups finely chopped baby spinach

½ cup finely chopped onion

1 tablespoon minced fresh ginger

1 tablespoon curry powder

½ teaspoon salt

¼ cup extra-virgin olive oil

1 (15-ounce) can chickpeas, rinsed

1 cup chopped zucchini

4 large eggs

Instructions:

Combine potatoes, spinach, onion, ginger, curry powder, and salt in a large bowl. Heat oil in a large nonstick skillet over medium-high heat. Add the potato mixture and press into a layer. Cook, without stirring, until crispy and golden brown on the bottom, 3 to 5 minutes.

Reduce heat to medium-low. Fold in chickpeas and zucchini, breaking up chunks of potato, until just combined. Press back into an even layer. Carve out 4 "wells" in the mixture. Break eggs, one at a time, into a cup and slip one into each indentation. Cover and continue cooking until the eggs are set, 4 to 5 minutes for soft-set yolks.

SNACK

carrot sticks and hummus

LUNCH

GREEK CHICKEN PASTA

PREP 15 min

COOK 15 min

READY IN 30 min

Ingredients:

Original recipe makes 6 servings

- 1 (16 ounce) package linguine pasta

- 1/2 cup chopped red onion

- 1 tablespoon olive oil

- 2 cloves garlic, crushed

- 1 pound skinless, boneless chicken breast meat–cut into bite-size pieces 2 lemons, wedged, for garnish

- 1 (14 ounce) can marinated artichoke hearts, drained and chopped

- 1 large tomato, chopped

- 1/2 cup crumbled feta cheese

- 3 tablespoons chopped fresh parsley

- 2 tablespoons lemon juice

- 2 teaspoons dried oregano

- salt and pepper to taste

Instructions:

- Bring a large pot of lightly salted water to a boil. Cook pasta in boiling water until tender yet firm to the bit, 8 to 10 minutes; drain.

- Heat olive oil in a large skillet over medium-high heat. Add onion and garlic: sauté until fragrant, about 2 minutes. Stir in the chicken and cook, stirring occasionally, until chicken is no longer pink in the center and the juices run clear, about 5 to 6 minutes.

Reduce heat to medium-low; add artichoke hearts, tomato, feta cheese, parsley, lemon juice, oregano, and cooked pasta. Cook and stir until heated through, about 2 to 3 minutes. Remove from heat, season with salt and pepper, and garnish with lemon wedges.

SNACK

1 cup Greek yogurt topped with nuts

DINNER

Mediterranean Seafood Grill with Skordalia

Ingredients:

- 1 pound russet or Yukon gold potatoes

- 8 garlic cloves, peeled

- 1 slice sourdough bread, crust removed

- 1/4 cup plain Greek low-fat yogurt

- 3 tablespoons olive oil, divided

- Zest and juice of 1 lemon

- 1/2 teaspoon salt, divided

- 1/4 teaspoon dried thyme

- 1 pound halibut fillets, cut into 4 pieces

- 2 red bell peppers, quartered

- 1 pound small zucchini, diagonally cut into 1-inch pieces

- 1/2 red onion, sliced

Instructions:

Peel potatoes, and chop into 1-inch pieces. Place in a large saucepan, and cover with cold water. Add garlic, and cook over high heat about 15 minutes or until potatoes are easily pierced with a fork.

While potatoes cook, tear bread into 3 or 4 pieces and place in a large bowl. Spoon 2 to 3 tablespoons cooking liquid from potatoes over bread. Stir with a fork until smooth. Add yogurt, 2 tablespoons olive oil, and zest and juice of 1 lemon; stir until a smooth paste forms.

When the potatoes are done, place a large bowl in the sink and set a colander on top. Drain potatoes and garlic, reserving cooking liquid. Transfer potatoes to bread mixture and mash until smooth (a potato ricer works well for this task). Add reserved cooking liquid 2 tablespoons at a time until mixture takes on the consistency of loose mashed potatoes. Stir in ½ teaspoon salt and 2 teaspoons olive oil. Cover and keep warm until ready to serve.

Preheat grill pan over medium-high heat. Drizzle fish with ½ teaspoon olive oil and season with remaining ½ teaspoon salt and thyme. Cook fish 2 to 3 minutes on each side until fish flakes when tested with a fork or until desired degree of doneness. Transfer to a plate; cover and keep warm until ready to serve.

Place bell pepper, zucchini, and red onion in a large bowl. Drizzle with remaining ½ teaspoon olive oil; toss to coat. Arrange bell pepper in grill pan and cook 5 minutes over medium heat. Add zucchini and onion; cook 10 minutes or until vegetables are tender, turning as necessary to ensure even cooking.

Calories per serving:	390
Fat per serving:	14g

BREAKFAST

Zucchini and Goat Cheese Frittata

Prep time: 30 minutes

Cook time: 20 minutes

Yield: 4 servings

Ingredients:

2 medium zucchinis

8 eggs

2 tablespoons milk

1/4 teaspoon salt

1/8 teaspoon pepper

1 tablespoon olive oil

1 clove garlic, crushed

2 ounces goat cheese, crumbled

- **Instructions:**

- Preheat the oven to 350 degrees. Slice the zucchinis into 1/4-inch-thick round slices. In a large bowl whisk the eggs with the milk, salt, and pepper.

- In a heavy, ovenproof skillet (preferably cast iron), heat the olive oil over medium heat. Add the garlic and cook for 30 seconds. Add the zucchini slices and cook for 5 minutes.

- Pour the whisked eggs over the zucchini and stir for 1 minute. Top with the cheese and transfer to the oven. Bake for 10 to 12 minutes or until the eggs are set. Remove the pan from the oven and let sit for 3 minutes.

- Transfer the frittata to a cutting board, slice into four pie wedges, and serve hot or at room temperature.

Per serving: Calories 134 (From Fat 72); Fat 8g (Saturated 3g); Cholesterol 11mg; Sodium 324mg; Carbohydrate 4g (Dietary Fiber 1g); Protein 12g.

SNACK

apple and ½ cup Greek yogurt

LUNCH

Zucchini Pie

Marjoram, with its hint of balsam, complements mild yellow and green summer squash in this simple crust less zucchini pie. It is topped by tomato slices and low-fat feta cheese, a lean choice. If yellow zucchini are unavailable, use all green zucchini.

Ingredients:

- 2 teaspoons olive oil

- 1 pound (about 2 or 3) green zucchini, cut into 1/2-inch pieces

- 4 scallions, thinly sliced

- 4 cloves garlic, minced

- 1 teaspoon dried marjoram

- 1 teaspoon coarse salt

- 1/2 teaspoon freshly ground pepper

- 1 pound (about 2 or 3) yellow zucchini, cut into 1/2-inch pieces

- 1/2 cup freshly chopped dill

- 1/4 cup freshly chopped flat-leaf parsley

- 5 large eggs plus 5 large egg whites, lightly beaten

- 1 tomato, thinly sliced

- 2 ounces low-fat feta cheese, crumbled

Instructions:

Preheat oven to 325 degrees. Heat 1 teaspoon olive oil in a large skillet set over medium heat. Add green zucchini, half the scallions, half the garlic, A teaspoon marjoram, 1/2 teaspoon salt, and 1/4 teaspoon pepper; cook, stirring frequently, until zucchini has softened and is beginning to brown, about 5 minutes. Remove from heat; transfer to a large bowl; set aside.

Rinse skillet; repeat process with yellow zucchini and remaining teaspoon olive oil, scallions, garlic, 1/2 teaspoon marjoram, 1/2 teaspoon salt, and 1/4 teaspoon pepper. Transfer to bowl with cooked green zucchini; let sit until cooled. Drain and discard any liquid.

Add dill, parsley, and eggs to zucchini; stir to combine. Pour into a 9 1/2-inch round, deep baking dish. Cover with tomato; sprinkle with feta. Bake until set, about 1 hour. Serve hot or at room temperature.

SNACK

1 cup almonds or walnuts

DINNER

Whole-Wheat Greek Pizza

- *Prep Time 10 minutes*

- *Total Time 30 minutes*

- *Yield Serves 4*

There's no need to buy a special pizza pan; an upside-down baking sheet works just as well. If you like, you can add a little cornmeal to the baking sheet before cooking.

Ingredients:

- 2 tablespoons olive oil, plus more for baking sheet

- 1 cup cherry tomatoes

- 1 clove garlic, coarsely chopped

- Coarse salt and freshly ground pepper

- Whole-wheat flour, for work surface

- 1 pound whole-wheat pizza dough, thawed if frozen

- 1 cup (4 ounces) grated cheese (mozzarella works best)

- 2 tablespoons pine nuts

- 2 cups baby arugula

- 1 tablespoon red-wine vinegar

- 1/4 cup pitted kalamata olives, coarsely chopped

Instructions:

- Preheat oven to 450 degrees. Turn a large baking sheet upside down; rub with oil. Place tomatoes, garlic, and 1 tablespoon oil in a food processor; season with salt and pepper. Pulse 3 to 4 times until ingredients are incorporated but chunky.

- On a lightly floured work surface, use a rolling pin and your hands to roll and stretch dough until large enough to cover the surface of the baking sheet. (If dough becomes too elastic, let it rest a few minutes.) Transfer to prepared baking sheet.

- Spread tomato sauce evenly over dough, leaving a 1-inch border all around. Top with cheese and pine nuts; season with salt and pepper.

Bake until crust is golden, 15 to 20 minutes. Toss arugula with vinegar and 1 tablespoon oil; season with salt and pepper. Sprinkle arugula and olives over pizza.

BREAKFAST

Savory Fava Beans with Warm Pita Bread

Prep time: 10 minutes

Cook time: 15 minutes

Yield: 4 servings

Ingredients:

1-1/2 tablespoons olive oil

1 large onion, chopped

1 large tomato, diced

1 clove garlic, crushed

One 15-ounce can fava beans, undrained

1 teaspoon ground cumin

1/4 cup chopped fresh parsley

1/4 cup lemon juice

Salt and pepper to taste

Crushed red pepper flakes, to taste

4 whole-grain pita bread pockets

Instructions:

- In a large nonstick skillet, heat the olive oil over medium-high heat for 30 seconds. Add the onion, tomato, and garlic and sauté for 3 minutes, until soft. Add the fava beans and their liquid and bring to a boil.

- Reduce the heat to medium and add the cumin, parsley, and lemon juice and season with the salt, pepper, and ground red pepper to taste. Cook for 5 minutes on medium heat.

- Meanwhile, heat the pita in a cast-iron skillet over medium-low heat until warm (1 to 2 minutes per side). Serve the warm pita with the fava beans (either on the side or loaded up with the bean mixture).

Per serving: Calories 325 (From Fat 64); Fat 7g (Saturated 1g); Cholesterol 0mg; Sodium 831mg; Carbohydrate 56g (Dietary Fiber 10g); Protein 13g.

SNACK

Greek yogurt

LUNCH

Chopped Greek Salad

Makes: 4 servings, about 3 cups each

Active Time: 25 minutes

Total Time: 25 minutes

Chicken turns this Greek-inspired salad into a substantial main course. Feel free to substitute other chopped fresh vegetables, such as broccoli or bell peppers, for the tomatoes or cucumber. Use leftover chicken, store-roasted chicken or quickly poach a couple boneless, skinless chicken breasts while you prepare the rest of the salad. Serve with pita bread and hummus.

Ingredients:

- 1/3 cup red-wine vinegar

- 2 tablespoons extra-virgin olive oil

- 1 tablespoon chopped fresh dill, or oregano or 1 teaspoon dried

- 1 teaspoon garlic powder

- 1/4 teaspoon salt

- 1/4 teaspoon freshly ground pepper

- 6 cups chopped romaine lettuce

- 2 1/2 cups chopped cooked chicken, (about 12 ounces; see Tip)

- 2 medium tomatoes, chopped

- 1 medium cucumber, peeled, seeded and chopped

- 1/2 cup finely chopped red onion

- 1/2 cup sliced ripe black olives

- 1/2 cup crumbled feta cheese

- **Instructions:**

Whisk vinegar, oil, dill (or oregano), garlic powder, salt and pepper in a large bowl. Add lettuce, chicken, tomatoes, cucumber, onion, olives and feta; toss to coat.

Tips and Notes:

- Tip: If you don't have cooked chicken, poach 1 pound chicken breasts for this recipe. Place boneless, skinless chicken breasts in a medium skillet or saucepan. Add lightly salted water (or chicken broth) to cover and bring to a boil. Cover, reduce heat to low and simmer gently until the chicken is cooked through and no longer pink in the middle, 10 to 15 minutes.

Nutrition:

Per serving: 343 calories; 18 g fat (5 g sat, 7 g mono); 89 mg cholesterol; 11 g carbohydrates; 31 g protein

DINNER

Turkey-Hummus Sliders

Ingredients:

1 cucumber, diced

1/2 cup crumbled feta cheese

2 tablespoons red wine vinegar

1 teaspoon dried mint

4 tablespoons extra-virgin olive oil

Kosher salt and freshly ground pepper

1 1/2 pounds ground turkey

1 cup hummus, preferably spicy or roasted red pepper (about a 7-ounce container)

1/2 cup chopped fresh parsley

2 teaspoons ground coriander

16 mini pita pockets, preferably whole wheat, split open and warmed

2 to 3 plum tomatoes, sliced

Instructions:

Toss the cucumber, feta, vinegar, mint, 1 tablespoon olive oil and a pinch each of salt and pepper in a bowl; cover and refrigerate.

Mix the turkey, 1/2 cup hummus, the parsley and coriander in a bowl; season generously with pepper. Dampen your hands and shape the mixture into 16 small patties, about 1/2 inch thick.

Heat 1 1/2 tablespoons olive oil in a medium cast-iron skillet over medium-high heat. Add half of the patties and cook until browned and cooked through, about 2 minutes per side. Transfer to a plate. Cook the remaining patties in the remaining 1 1/2 tablespoons olive oil.

Mix the remaining 1/2 cup hummus with a splash of hot water in a bowl. Spread some of the hummus on the inside of each pita; fill with a tomato slice, turkey patty and some of the cucumber mixture.

Nutritional Analysis

Per Serving

Calories 214

BREAKFAST

Mediterranean Breakfast Couscous

Rethink couscous with a bit of brown sugar and dried fruit, you can bring the whole grain to your Mediterranean diet. It makes about 4 servings.

Ingredients:

3 cups 1 percent low-fat milk

1 (2-inch) cinnamon stick

1 cup uncooked whole-wheat couscous

½ cup chopped dried apricots

¼ cup dried currants

6 teaspoons dark brown sugar, divided

¼ teaspoon salt

4 teaspoons butter, melted and divided

Instructions:

Combine milk and cinnamon stick in a large saucepan over medium-high heat; heat 3 minutes or until small bubbles form around inner edge of pot (about 180 degrees Fahrenheit.) Do not boil. Remove from heat; stir in couscous, apricots, currants, 4 teaspoons brown sugar, and salt. Cover the mixture, and let it stand 15 minutes.

Remove and discard cinnamon stick. Divide couscous among each of 4 bowls, and top each with 1 teaspoon melted butter and ½ teaspoon brown sugar. Serve immediately.

SNACK

fruit drizzled with honey or agave

LUNCH

Chicken, Broccoli Rabe & Feta on Toast

From Eating Well: The assertive flavor of broccoli rabe can be overpowering in dishes. But here, the sweet tomatoes and briny feta stand up to its bite, rendering this dish a rustic but comforting favorite. Still, if broccoli rabe proves too strong for your taste, you can substitute broccolini or even tiny, trimmed broccoli florets.

Ingredients:

- 4 thick slices whole-wheat country bread

- 1 clove garlic, peeled (optional), plus 1/4 cup chopped garlic

- 4 teaspoons extra-virgin olive oil, divided

- 1 pound chicken tenders, cut crosswise into 1/2-inch pieces

- 1 bunch broccoli rabe, stems trimmed, cut into 1-inch pieces, or 2 bunches broccolini, chopped

- 2 cups cherry tomatoes, halved

- 1 tablespoon red-wine vinegar

- 1/8 teaspoon salt

- Freshly ground pepper, to taste

- 3/4 cup crumbled feta cheese

Instructions:

- Grill or toast bread. Lightly rub with peeled garlic clove, if desired. Discard the garlic.

- Heat 2 teaspoons oil in a large nonstick skillet over high heat until shimmering but not smoking. Add chicken: cook, stirring occasionally, until just cooked through and no longer pink in the middle, 4 to 5 minutes. Transfer the chicken and any juices to a plate: cover to keep warm.

- Add the remaining 2 teaspoons oil to the pan. Add chopped garlic and cook, stirring constantly, until fragrant but not brown, about 30 seconds. Add broccoli rabe (or broccolini) and cook, stirring often, until bright green and just wilted, 2 to 4 minutes. Stir in tomatoes, vinegar, salt and pepper; cook, stirring occasionally, until the tomatoes are beginning to break down, 2 to 4 minutes. Return the chicken and juices to the pan, add feta cheese and stir to combine. Cook until heated through, 1 to 2 minutes. Serve warm over garlic toasts.

- **Tips and Notes:**

- Ingredient Note: Pleasantly pungent and mildly bitter, broccoli rabe, or rapini, is a member of the cabbage family and commonly used in Mediterranean cooking. Broccolini (a cross between broccoli and Chinese kale) is sweet and tender–the florets and stalks are edible.

Nutrition:

Per serving: 313 calories; 11 g fat (5 g sat, 5 g mono); 85 mg cholesterol; 26 g carbohydrates; 35 g protein; 4 g fiber; 653 mg sodium; 423 mg potassium.

Nutrition Bonus: Vitamin C (160% daily value), Vitamin A (140% dv), Selenium (28% dv), Calcium (20% dv).

Carbohydrate Servings: 2

Exchanges: 1 starch, 2 vegetable, 4 lean meat

SNACK

cucumbers, carrots & hummus

Dinner

Cube Steak Milanese

From Eating Well: The economical cube steak is elevated to new heights in this recipe. The salad, with chopped arugula, basil, tomatoes, onion and sharp Italian cheese, is the picture of summer simplicity; all it needs is olive oil and lemon to dress it.

Makes: 4 servings, 1 steak & 1 1/2 cups salad each

Active Time: 45 minutes

Total Time: 45 minutes

Ingredients:

- 4 plum tomatoes, seeded and chopped

- 1/2 cup diced red onion

- 1/2 teaspoon salt, divided

- 1 egg, plus 1 egg white

- 1/2 cup plain dry breadcrumbs

- 1/4 cup grated Pecorino Romano, or Parmesan cheese plus 1/4 cup shaved (see Tip), divided

- 2 tablespoons minced fresh parsley, (optional)

- 1 pound cube steak, cut into 4 portions

- 1/2 teaspoon freshly ground pepper, divided

- 6 teaspoons extra-virgin olive oil, divided

- 4 cups baby arugula, chopped

- 3/4 cup thinly sliced fresh basil leaves

- 1 tablespoon fresh lemon juice, plus lemon wedges for garnish

Instructions:

Combine tomatoes, onion and 1/4 teaspoon salt in a large bowl.

Whisk egg and egg white in a shallow dish. Combine breadcrumbs, grated cheese and parsley (if using) in another shallow dish. Season steak with the remaining 1/4 teaspoon salt and 1/4 teaspoon pepper. Dip each piece into the egg, allowing excess to drip off into the dish, then dip in the breadcrumb mixture and turn to coat.

Heat 2 teaspoons oil in a large nonstick skillet over medium heat. Add the steaks and cook until golden brown on the first side, about 3 minutes. Turn the steaks over, add 1 teaspoon oil and cook until the steaks are cooked through, 3 to 4 minutes more. Transfer to a plate; tent with foil to keep warm.

Add 1/4 cup shaved cheese to the tomato mixture. Add the remaining 1/4 teaspoon pepper, the remaining 3 teaspoons oil, arugula, basil and lemon juice; toss to combine. Serve the steaks on beds of the arugula-tomato salad. Garnish with lemon wedges.

- **Tips:**

- Use a vegetable peeler to shave hard Italian cheese, such as Parmesan or Pecorino Romano.

Nutrition:

Per serving: 348 calories; 17 g fat (5 g sat, 6 g mono); 130 mg cholesterol; 14 g carbohydrates; 35 g protein; 2 g fiber; 581 mg sodium; 339 mg potassium.

This is just a week meal plan. The entire book has plenty of easy, healthy recipes to choose from, and you can add a side dish and dessert to your dinner. For more recipe ideas to make your meal planning a cinch, check out the book.

BREAKFAST

Mediterranean Vegetable Omelet

Prep time: 15 minutes

Cook time: 25 minutes

Yield: 4 servings

Ingredients:

1 tablespoon olive oil

2 cups thinly sliced fresh fennel bulb

1 Roma tomato, diced

1/4 cup pitted green brine-cured olives, chopped

1/4 cup artichoke hearts, marinated in water, rinsed, drained, and chopped

6 eggs

1/4 teaspoon salt

1/2 teaspoon pepper

1/2 cup goat cheese, crumbled

2 tablespoons chopped fresh dill, basil, or parsley

- **Instructions:**

- Preheat the oven to 325 degrees. In a large ovenproof skillet, heat the olive oil over medium-high heat. Add the fennel and sauté for 5 minutes, until soft.

- Add in the tomato, olives, and artichoke hearts and sauté for 3 minutes, until softened.

- Whisk the eggs in a large bowl and season with the salt and pepper. Pour the whisked eggs into the skillet over the vegetables and stir with a heat-proof spoon for 2 minutes.

- Sprinkle the omelet with the cheese and bake for 5 minutes or until the eggs are cooked through and set.

- Top with the dill, basil, or parsley. Remove the omelet from the skillet onto a cutting board. Carefully cut the omelet into four wedges, like a pizza, and serve.

Per serving: Calories 152 (From Fat 91); Fat 10g (Saturated 4g); Cholesterol 13mg; Sodium 496mg; Carbohydrate 6g (Dietary Fiber 2g); Protein 11g.

Zucchini and Goat Cheese Frittata

Prep time: 30 minutes

Cook time: 20 minutes

Yield: 4 servings

Ingredients:

2 medium zucchinis

8 eggs

2 tablespoons milk

1/4 teaspoon salt

1/8 teaspoon pepper

1 tablespoon olive oil

1 clove garlic, crushed

2 ounces goat cheese, crumbled

- **Instructions:**

- Preheat the oven to 350 degrees. Slice the zucchinis into 1/4-inch-thick round slices. In a large bowl whisk the eggs with the milk, salt, and pepper.

- In a heavy, ovenproof skillet (preferably cast iron), heat the olive oil over medium heat. Add the garlic and cook for 30 seconds. Add the zucchini slices and cook for 5 minutes.

- Pour the whisked eggs over the zucchini and stir for 1 minute. Top with the cheese and transfer to the oven. Bake for 10 to 12 minutes or until the eggs are set. Remove the pan from the oven and let sit for 3 minutes.

- Transfer the frittata to a cutting board, slice into four pie wedges, and serve hot or at room temperature.

Per serving: Calories 134 (From Fat 72); Fat 8g (Saturated 3g); Cholesterol 11mg; Sodium 324mg; Carbohydrate 4g (Dietary Fiber 1g); Protein 12g.

Mediterranean Egg Scramble

Prep time: 15 minutes

Cook time: 25 minutes

Yield: 4 servings

Ingredients:

1 teaspoon olive oil

1 teaspoon butter

3 medium-sized new potatoes, thinly sliced

1/4 large red bell pepper, small diced

8 black olives, chopped

1/4 cup fresh parsley, chopped

1/4 cup fresh ricotta cheese

6 eggs

Salt and pepper to taste

4 slices crusty bread

4 teaspoons butter or extra-virgin olive oil

- **Instructions:**

- In a large nonstick skillet, heat the olive oil and butter to medium-high heat. Add the sliced potatoes and sauté for about 15 minutes or until golden. Add the bell pepper and olives and cook for 4 minutes.

- In a medium bowl, whisk together the parsley, ricotta, and eggs. Pour the egg mixture over the potato mixture, stirring every 30 seconds until firm and set but not dry, about 3 minutes. Salt and pepper the egg scramble to taste.

- Serve with crusty bread, lightly toasted and buttered with 1 teaspoon of butter or lightly brushed with 1 teaspoon of extra-virgin olive oil per slice.

Per serving: Calories 330 (From Fat 113); Fat 13g (Saturated 3g); Cholesterol 9mg; Sodium 364mg; Carbohydrate 43g (Dietary Fiber 4g); Protein 13g.

Lemon Scones

Prep time: 15 minutes

Cook time: 15 minutes

Yield: 12 servings

Ingredients:

2 cups plus 1/4 cup flour

2 tablespoons sugar

1/2 teaspoon baking soda

1/2 teaspoon salt

1/4 cup butter

Zest of one lemon

3/4 cup reduced fat buttermilk

1 cup powdered sugar

1 to 2 teaspoons lemon juice

Instructions:

- Heat the oven to 400 degrees. In a medium bowl, combine 2 cups of the flour, the sugar, baking soda, and salt. Using a pastry blender or a food processor, cut in the butter until the mixture resembles fine crumbs.

- Add the lemon zest and buttermilk, stirring just until mixed. Flour a surface with the remaining flour and turn out the dough; knead gently six times. Shape the dough into a ball and then flatten into a 1/2-inch-thick circle with a rolling pin.

- Cut the circle into 4 wedges and then cut each wedge into 3 smaller wedges, yielding 12 scones. Place the scones on baking sheet and cook for 12 to 15 minutes or until golden brown.

- In a small bowl, mix the powder sugar and just enough lemon juice to make a thin frosting. Drizzle the frosting over the hot scones and serve.

Per serving: Calories 175

(From Fat 39); Fat 4g (Saturated 3g); Cholesterol 11mg; Sodium 190mg; Carbohydrate 31g (Dietary Fiber 1g); Protein 3g.

Savory Fava Beans with Warm Pita Bread

Prep time: 10 minutes

Cook time: 15 minutes

Yield: 4 servings

Ingredients:

1-1/2 tablespoons olive oil

1 large onion, chopped

1 large tomato, diced

1 clove garlic, crushed

One 15-ounce can fava beans, undrained

1 teaspoon ground cumin

1/4 cup chopped fresh parsley

1/4 cup lemon juice

Salt and pepper to taste

Crushed red pepper flakes, to taste

4 whole-grain pita bread pockets

- **Instructions:**

- In a large nonstick skillet, heat the olive oil over medium-high heat for 30 seconds. Add the onion, tomato, and garlic and sauté for 3 minutes, until soft. Add the fava beans and their liquid and bring to a boil.

- Reduce the heat to medium and add the cumin, parsley, and lemon juice and season with the salt, pepper, and ground red pepper to taste. Cook for 5 minutes on medium heat.

- Meanwhile, heat the pita in a cast-iron skillet over medium-low heat until warm (1 to 2 minutes per side). Serve the warm pita with the fava beans (either on the side or loaded up with the bean mixture).

- *Per serving: Calories 325 (From Fat 64); Fat 7g (Saturated 1g); Cholesterol 0mg; Sodium 831mg; Carbohydrate 56g (Dietary Fiber 10g); Protein 13g.*

Mediterranean Breakfast Couscous

Heath.com

Rethink couscous with a bit of brown sugar and dried fruit, you can bring the whole grain to your Mediterranean diet. It makes about 4 servings.

Ingredients:

3 cups 1 percent low-fat milk

1 (2-inch) cinnamon stick

1 cup uncooked whole-wheat couscous

½ cup chopped dried apricots

¼ cup dried currants

6 teaspoons dark brown sugar, divided

¼ teaspoon salt

4 teaspoons butter, melted and divided

Instructions:

Combine milk and cinnamon stick in a large saucepan over medium-high heat; heat 3 minutes or until small bubbles form around inner edge of pot (about 180 degrees Fahrenheit.) Do not boil. Remove from heat; stir in couscous, apricots, currants, 4 teaspoons brown sugar, and salt. Cover the mixture, and let it stand 15 minutes. Remove and discard cinnamon stick. Divide couscous among each of 4 bowls, and top each with 1 teaspoon melted butter and ½ teaspoon brown sugar. Serve immediately.

Chickpea and Potato Hash

Eating Well

This hash will be a suitable meal choice anytime of the day, including breakfast. It will certainly keep you full, containing 14 grams of protein, and 6 grams of fiber per serving; it will make enough for 4 people.

Ingredients:

4 cups frozen shredded hash brown potatoes

2 cups finely chopped baby spinach

½ cup finely chopped onion

1 tablespoon minced fresh ginger

1 tablespoon curry powder

½ teaspoon salt

¼ cup extra-virgin olive oil

1 (15-ounce) can chickpeas, rinsed

1 cup chopped zucchini

4 large eggs

Instructions:

Combine potatoes, spinach, onion, ginger, curry powder, and salt in a large bowl. Heat oil in a large nonstick skillet over medium-high heat.

Add the potato mixture and press into a layer. Cook, without stirring, until crispy and golden brown on the bottom, 3 to 5 minutes.

Reduce heat to medium-low. Fold in chickpeas and zucchini, breaking up chunks of potato, until just combined. Press back into an even layer. Carve out 4 "wells" in the mixture. Break eggs, one at a time, into a cup and slip one into each indentation. Cover and continue cooking until the eggs are set, 4 to 5 minutes for soft-set yolks.

Pancakes

Get a side of whole grains with your Greek yogurt by making a stack of pancakes using the recipe from Oikos. Top them off with fresh fruit, toasted nuts, more Greek yogurt, or sweeten the stack with a dash of syrup. It makes about 6 servings.

.

Ingredients:

1 cup old-fashioned oats

½ cup all purpose whole wheat flour

2 tablespoons flax seeds

1 teaspoon baking soda

¼ teaspoon salt

2 cups Greek yogurt (plain or vanilla)

2 large eggs

2 tablespoons agave or honey

2 tablespoons canola oil

syrup, fresh fruit, or other toppings

Instructions:

Combine first five ingredients in a blender and pulse process 30 seconds. Add yogurt, eggs, oil, and agave and blend until smooth.

Let batter stand to thicken, about 20 minutes. (Batter can be prepared up to 1 day in advance; cover batter and refrigerate.)

Heat large non-stick skillet over medium heat. Brush skillet with oil.

Working in batches, ladle batter by ¼ cupful into skillet. Cook pancakes until bottoms are golden brown and bubbles form on top, about 2 minutes. Turn pancakes over; cook until bottoms are golden brown, about 2 minutes. Transfer to baking sheet. Keep warm in oven. Repeat with remaining batter, brushing skillet with more butter as necessary. Serve with desired toppings.

Banana Nut Oatmeal

You can use walnuts or almonds to top off a bowl of oatmeal in this AllRecipes.com oatmeal.

Ingredients:

¼ cup quick cooking oats

½ cup skim milk

1 teaspoon flax seeds

2 tablespoons chopped walnuts

3 tablespoons honey

1 banana, peeled

Instructions:

Combine the oats, milk, flax seeds, walnuts, honey, and banana in a microwave-safe bowl. Cook in microwave on High for 2 minutes. Mash the banana with a fork and stir into the mixture. Serve hot.

SNACK IDEAS

#1 Chickpeas roasted with olive oil, salt and paprika

It is possible to have a satisfyingly crunchy and salty snack without reaching for a bag of chips. Make your own spiced, roasted chickpeas: Rinse, drain and pat dry two cans of chickpeas. Place them on a rimmed baking sheet, and drizzle them with olive oil. Roast in a hot oven until dark and crunchy, 30 to 40 minutes. Sprinkle with salt and paprika to taste, and roast a few minutes more. Chickpeas and olive oil are staples of the Mediterranean diet; the beans are rich in fiber, and olive oil delivers heart-healthy monounsaturated fat. (And even your favorite picky eater will love them.)

#2 Baked sweet potato fries made with olive oil

Not all comfort food is bad for you. Sweet potatoes are a nutritional powerhouse — so much so that the nutrition scientists at the Center for Science in the Public Interest (CSPI) rank the orange tuber number-one in good-for-you vegetables. The reason? For starters, they're loaded with carotenoids, antioxidants that have been associated with a lower risk of death from heart disease, cancer and other diseases. Sweet potatoes are also chock-full of fiber, which helps keep their glycemic index lower than all other root vegetables. Indulge guilt-free by making baked sweet potato fries. Slice potatoes length-wise into half-inch-wide blocks. Toss in a bowl with olive oil, salt and pepper (you can also add other spices, like cayenne pepper or basil), and lay in a single layer on a foil-covered cookie sheet. Bake at 425 degrees for 30 minutes, flipping them every 10 minutes.

#3 Kumquats

If you love tart apples or foods that make you pucker, pick up a pint of kumquats next time you're at the supermarket. About an inch tall, the citrusy fruit looks like a miniature orange. The only difference is, you eat the whole thing, rind and all. You can swallow the seeds or spit them out (depending on your company). While the fruit's skin is sweet, the interior pulp packs a mouth-puckering zing. One serving of kumquats (about seven of them) has 90 calories, 9 grams of fiber and 3 grams of protein. It will also give you your day's worth of vitamin C, plus a moderate amount of vitamin A, calcium and iron. Unlike your typical juicy orange, kumquats make for a mess-free on-the-go snack. Eat alone; slice and add to a salad with goat cheese, chopped apples, dried cranberries and nuts; or chop and add to a mango salsa that you can serve over salmon.

#4 Plain Greek yogurt

Looking for a healthful, creamy snack? Look no further than Greek yogurt. Unlike regular plain yogurt, Greek yogurt is thick, rich and tangy. It tastes delicious with fresh or dried fruit or cinnamon added, and Greek yogurt is a protein powerhouse. A six-ounce container of one brand, Fage 0% fat yogurt, contains 18 grams of protein (the amount you'll get in three eggs, but with none of the saturated fat or cholesterol). Not only is it a terrific stand alone snack, it's also one of our favorite additions to a variety of meals, like a topping for a spicy black bean and brown rice burrito. Yum!

#5 Dried apples

There's no bad apple in this bunch! According to a study presented at the annual Federation of the American Societies for

Experimental Biology meeting, women who snacked on dried apples every day earned a bushel of heart-healthy benefits. Those who ate 240 calories worth of dried apples for a year lowered their "lousy" LDL cholesterol by 23 percent. It also reduced levels of C-reactive protein and lipid hydroperoxide — two substances linked with an increased risk of heart disease. Women who grazed on the dried fruit also whittled their waist, losing an average of 3.3 pounds over the course of the year. Since the average 140-pound woman gains 1.3 pounds per year, that's like shaving almost five pounds off your frame, just by eating apples. Although the reason for this effect is not exactly known, apples are a great source of fiber, which can both fill you up and whisk cholesterol out of your bloodstream. They also contain chemicals called polyphenols, which have been shown to affect the way cholesterol is made in the body, as well as how fat around the middle is affected. Just remember to choose the unsweetened variety. Arrange them on a cookie sheet lined with parchment paper, and sprinkle with cinnamon, if desired. Put them in the oven for up to two hours at 200 degrees. Depending on how thick your apple slices are, they may brown quickly, so keep a close eye on them so they don't burn. The apple chips, slightly chewy when removed from the oven, will turn crispy as they cool.

#6 Pistachios

Looking for a snack that's filling and kind to your waistline? Treat yourself to a handful of pistachios — the so-called skinny nut. Out of all nuts, pistachios have the fewest calories — just 160 per one-ounce serving (about 50 nuts). This "skinny nut" is also packed with the same antioxidants found in other nuts such as walnuts and almonds. A new USDA study found that the fat in pistachios may not be completely absorbed by the body, which means they could have even less than 160 calories per serving. More research is needed to tell for sure. Still, because you have to pry them out of their shells, pistachios take longer to eat than other snacks and tend to discourage overeating. In fact, research shows that snackers consume 41 percent fewer calories when eating pistachios over other, already-shelled nuts. The ever-growing pile of discarded shells also helps us better visualize how much we've already eaten, so we'll be less likely to mindlessly devour the entire bag.

#7 Medjool dates

Got a serious sweet tooth? You don't need a brownie or candy bar to get your sugar fix. Indulge in a couple of Medjool dates instead.

These large, moist delicacies are tender and sticky with a sweet caramel taste. A two-date snack (which, believe us, is all you'll need) will set you back about 140 calories. One serving packs 4 grams of fiber and 10 percent of your daily potassium needs. And, despite their sugar content, antioxidant-rich dates do not appear to have negative effects on triglycerides or blood sugar levels, according to a study in the Journal of Agricultural and Food Chemistry. Eat them alone, or add them, chopped, to a salad with kumquats and goat cheese for a sweet-tart flavor combination.

#8 Pumpkin Seeds

Pumpkin seeds are a good source of the amino acid tryptophan, which the body uses to manufacture serotonin, a hormone associated with improved mood and sleep. Roast them yourself by buying raw pumpkin seeds (sometimes called pepitas), spreading them on a rimmed baking sheet, drizzling with olive oil and seasoning with a bit of salt and pepper. Bake in a 350-degree oven for approximately 15 minutes, stirring occasionally. Snack on a handful of them in mid-morning or during the afternoon. Or sprinkle pumpkin seeds on yogurt, over salads, or on top of baked sweet potatoes.

#9 Hummus Dip

Hummus, made from a base of chickpeas and olive oil, is a tasty and healthy snack — great for parties or keeping stocked in your refrigerator as a dip for cut veggies or whole-grain pita.

#10 Healthy banana "gelato"

If ice cream is your go-to treat when you're craving something sweet, try this guilt-free version instead: frozen blended bananas. Whipping frozen bananas in a blender turns them into a thick, rich, custardy treat. Here's how: Peel and slice a couple of ripened bananas. Place them on a cookie sheet in a single layer and freeze for two hours. Blend the fruit in a food processor or blender, scraping the mixture off the sides when it sticks, until it has a smooth, custardy consistency. Serve immediately. Experiment with different flavors by adding in peanut butter, hazelnut butter or fresh berries. You'll be amazed by just how good something so simple can be. Eat it plain or spread over graham crackers for an open-faced ice cream sandwich.

Adapted ideas from cleavelandclinicwellness.com

SOUPS AND SALADS

Mediterranean Red Lentil Bean Soup

Ingredients:

- 2 tablespoons extra virgin olive oil

- 2 large onions–diced

- 8 cups of stock–chicken or vegetable

- 2 cups dried red lentil beans–rinsed and sorted

- 2 ripe tomatoes–cubed

- 1 teaspoon ground cumin

- Salt and pepper to taste

- 1–2 finely chopped carrots (optional)

- 2 cups fresh spinach (optional)

- ½ raw potato–grated (optional)

Instructions:

- Soak the lentils for a few hours and throw away the water. Boil the lentils until they are half cooked (the cooking time depends on the size and type of lentil). Taste one to see if it is approximately half cooked. Heat the olive oil in a soup pot. Sauté the diced onions (and carrots if desired) in the olive oil. Place the tomatoes, stock and (spinach and/or potato if desired) into the pot. Add cumin, salt and pepper. Add any additional seasonings desired. Simmer for approximately 30 to 40 minutes or until the lentils are tender. Add water as necessary. Add a dash of olive oil just before serving.

Fish Soup with Rotelle

Ingredients:

- 2 tablespoons extra virgin olive oil

- 1 onion, diced

- 1 tablespoon minced garlic

- ½ can crushed tomatoes

- 1 cup Rotelle (round pasta)

- 1 dozen mussels in their shells

- 1 pound monkfish

- ¼ teaspoon rosemary

Instructions:

- Sauté the onion and garlic in the olive oil until soft. Add one quart water, the tomatoes, rosemary and pasta. Add salt and pepper to taste and cook for 15 minutes. Clean the mussels well and cut the fish into bite-sized pieces. Add to the soup and simmer for another 10 minutes. All of the mussel shells should be open at this point. Discard any unopened ones. Serve with crusty bread and olive oil.

Minestrone

Prep time: 15 minutes

Cook time: 6–8 hours

Yield: 8 servings

Ingredients:

1 onion, diced

3 carrots, washed, quartered and sliced into 1/2-inch slices

3 celery stalks, quartered and sliced into 1/2-inch slices

Two 14.5-ounce cans navy beans, drained and rinsed

One 28-ounce can diced tomatoes

4 cups low-sodium chicken stock

4 Italian chicken sausage links, quartered and sliced into 1/2-inch slices

2 sprigs thyme, or 1/2 teaspoon dried thyme

2 bay leaves

1/2 teaspoon dried sage

1 cup orzo or other small pasta

3 zucchinis, quartered and sliced into 1/2-inch slices

1/2 cup freshly grated Parmesan for serving

Salt to taste (optional)

- **Instructions:**

- Stir the onions, carrots, celery, beans, tomatoes, stock, sausage, thyme, bay leaves, and sage together in a 4- to 5-quart slow cooker. Cook on low for 6 to 8 hours. During the last 30 minutes of cooking, add the orzo and zucchini and cook for 30 minutes on high or until you're ready to serve. Add salt to taste (if desired). Divide the soup among eight bowls, removing the bay leaves. Top each bowl with 1 tablespoon of the grated Parmesan and serve.

Per serving: Calories 382 (From Fat 98); Fat 11g (Saturated 4g); Cholesterol 25mg; Sodium 1178mg; Carbohydrate 50g (Dietary Fiber 10g); Protein 23g.

Cabbage and Bean Soup

Prep time: 10 minutes

Cook time: 50 minutes

Yield: 6 servings

Ingredients:

1/4 cup olive oil

1 medium onion, chopped

2 carrots, chopped

2 celery stalks, chopped

6 sprigs parsley

1 bay leaf

1/4 teaspoon dried sage

One 14.5-ounce can diced tomatoes

8 cups water

1/2 pound Yukon gold potatoes, cut into bite-sized pieces

1 pound green cabbage, chopped (about 6 cups)

1/2 pound baked ham, cut into 1-inch cubes

One 14.5-ounce can cannellini beans, drained

1/4 cup instant polenta

Salt and pepper to taste

- **Instructions:**

- Heat the olive oil in a large stock pot over medium heat for 1 minute. Add the onions, carrots, and celery and cook until the onions are translucent, about 6 to 7 minutes.

- Add the tomatoes (with juice), parsley, bay leaf, and sage; lower the heat to low and simmer for 10 minutes.

- Raise the heat to medium-high, add the water, and bring the mixture to a boil. Add the potatoes, cabbage, ham, and beans. Cover and drop the heat to simmer for 20 minutes or until the potatoes are tender.

- Whisk in the polenta and continue whisking for 4 to 5 minutes. Season with salt and pepper. Serve.

Per serving: Calories 345 (From Fat 110); Fat 12g (Saturated 2g);

Cholesterol 21mg; Sodium 754mg; Carbohydrate 44g (Dietary Fiber

Pasta Fagioli

Prep time: 10 minutes

Cook time: 30 minutes

Yield: 8 servings

Ingredients:

1 tablespoon olive oil

2 ounces pancetta, diced small

1 teaspoon dried rosemary, minced

1/2 teaspoon dried thyme, or 2 sprigs fresh thyme

1 bay leaf

1/4 teaspoon red pepper flakes

1 medium onion, chopped small

2 medium carrots, diced small

2 celery stalks, diced small

6 cloves garlic, sliced

Two 14.5-ounce cans cannellini or navy beans, drained and rinsed

One 14.5-ounce can diced tomatoes, undrained

8 cups low-sodium chicken or vegetable stock

2 inches Parmesan rind (optional)

1 cup ditalini or other small pasta

Salt and pepper to taste

1/2 cup freshly grated Parmesan cheese

- **Instructions:**

- In a large stock pot, heat the olive oil over medium heat for 2 minutes. Add the pancetta and sauté for 3 to 5 minutes. Add the rosemary, thyme, bay leaf, red pepper flakes, onions, carrots, celery, and garlic.

- Continue to sauté for 7 minutes or until the onions are translucent. Add the beans, tomatoes (juice included), and stock. Bring soup to a boil and lower the heat to simmer.

- Add the Parmesan rind (if desired) and pasta and continue to cook for 20 minutes or until the pasta and vegetables are tender. Remove the rind and discard.

- Season the soup with salt and pepper. Serve each bowl with 1 tablespoon of freshly grated Parmesan cheese.

Per serving: Calories 290 (From Fat 60); Fat 7g (Saturated 2g); Cholesterol 8mg; Sodium 796mg; Carbohydrate 42g (Dietary Fiber 7g); Protein 18g.

Mediterranean Kale, Cannellini and Farro Stew

Prep Time: 15 minutes

Cook Time: 40 minutes

Yield: 6 servings

Ingredients:

- 2 Tbsp olive oil

- 1 cup carrots diced (about 2 medium)

- 1 cup chopped yellow onion (1 small)

- 1 cup chopped celery (about 2)

- 4 cloves garlic, minced

- 1 (32 oz) carton low-sodium vegetable broth

- 1 (15 oz) can diced tomatoes

- 1 cup farro, rinsed

- 1 tsp dried oregano

- 1 bay leaf

- Salt, to taste

- 1/2 cup slightly packed parsley sprigs (stems included)

- 4 cups slightly packed chopped kale, thick ribs removed

- 1 (15 oz) can cannellini beans, drained and rinsed

- 3 teaspoons fresh lemon juice

- Feta cheese, crumbled, for serving

- **Instructions:**

- Heat oil in a large pot over medium-high heat. Add carrots, onion and celery and saute 3 minutes. Add garlic and saute 30 seconds longer. Stir in vegetable broth, tomatoes, farro, oregano, bay leaf and season with salt to taste. Lay parsley in a mound on top of soup and bring soup to a boil. Reduce heat just below medium. Cover and cook 20 minutes, then remove parsley, stir in kale and cook 10–15 minutes longer, adding in cannellini beans during last few minutes of cooking, until both farro and kale are tender.

Remove bay leaf, stir in lemon juice and add additional vegetable broth or some water to thin soup as desired (the farro will absorb more liquid as the soup rests). Serve warm topping each serving with feta cheese.

Orange, Anchovy & Olive Salad

From Eating Well

This delightful Italian salad recipe brings together oranges, olives and anchovies. Beautiful and refreshing, this simple salad can easily be made ahead. Serve as a first course or with roasted chicken.

Ingredients:

- 4 small oranges, preferably blood oranges

- 1 small red onion, sliced into very thin rounds

- 16 salt-cured (or oil-cured) black olives or Kalamata olives, pitted and halved

- 6 anchovy fillets

- 1 tablespoon fresh lemon juice

- 3 tablespoons extra-virgin olive oil

- 1/8 teaspoon ground pepper, or more to taste

- 2 teaspoons finely minced fennel fronds for garnish

- **Instructions:**

Peel oranges carefully with a paring knife, cutting away all the white pith as well as the membrane that covers them on the outside. Working on a plate to help capture all the juice, slice the oranges into rounds, as thin as you can manage.

Arrange the orange slices on a serving platter; reserve the juice. Distribute onion over the oranges, then arrange olives over the top and finally the anchovy fillets.

Pour the orange juice and lemon juice over the salad and drizzle with oil. Sprinkle with pepper.

Let the salad stand at room temperature for about 30 minutes to let the flavors develop. Serve sprinkled with fennel fronds, if desired.

Nutrition:

Per serving: 202 calories; 15 g fat (2 g sat, 11 g mono); 5 mg cholesterol; 15 g carbohydrates; 0 g added sugars; 2 g total sugars; 3 g protein; 3 g fiber; 465 mg sodium; 237 mg potassium.

Nutrition Bonus: Vitamin C (90% daily value)

Carbohydrate Servings: 1

Exchanges: 1 fruit, 1/2 vegetable, 3 fat

Caprese Salad

- *PREP 15 mins*

- *READY IN 15 mins*

Ingredients:

Original recipe makes 6 servings

- 4 large ripe tomatoes, sliced 1/4 inch thick

- 1 pound fresh mozzarella cheese, sliced 1/4 inch thick

- 1/3 cup fresh basil leaves

- 3 tablespoons extra virgin olive oil

- fine sea salt to taste

- freshly ground black pepper to taste

- **Instructions:**

On a large platter, alternate and overlap the tomato slices, mozzarella cheese slices, and basil leaves. Drizzle with olive oil. Season with sea salt and pepper.

Chopped Greek Salad with Chicken

Makes: 4 servings, about 3 cups each

Active Time: 25 minutes

Total Time: 25 minutes

From Eating Well

Chicken turns this Greek-inspired salad into a substantial main course. Feel free to substitute other chopped fresh vegetables, such as broccoli or bell peppers, for the tomatoes or cucumber. Use leftover chicken, store-roasted chicken or quickly poach a couple boneless, skinless chicken breasts while you prepare the rest of the salad. Serve with pita bread and hummus.

Ingredients:

- 1/3 cup red-wine vinegar

- 2 tablespoons extra-virgin olive oil

- 1 tablespoon chopped fresh dill, or oregano or 1 teaspoon dried

- 1 teaspoon garlic powder

- 1/4 teaspoon salt

- 1/4 teaspoon freshly ground pepper

- 6 cups chopped romaine lettuce

- 2 1/2 cups chopped cooked chicken, (about 12 ounces; see Tip)

- 2 medium tomatoes, chopped

- 1 medium cucumber, peeled, seeded and chopped

- 1/2 cup finely chopped red onion

- 1/2 cup sliced ripe black olives

- 1/2 cup crumbled feta cheese

- **Instructions:**

Whisk vinegar, oil, dill (or oregano), garlic powder, salt and pepper in a large bowl. Add lettuce, chicken, tomatoes, cucumber, onion, olives and feta; toss to coat.

Nutrition:

Per serving: 343 calories; 18 g fat (5 g sat, 7 g mono); 89 mg cholesterol; 11 g carbohydrates; 31 g protein; 3 g fiber; 619 mg sodium; 659 mg potassium.

Nutrition Bonus: Vitamin A (140% daily value), Vitamin C (45% dv), Folate (31% dv), Potassium (19% dv), Calcium (15% dv).

Carbohydrate Servings: 1

Exchanges: 2 vegetable, 3 1/2 lean meat, 2 fat

Easy Arugula Salad

Ingredients:

- 4 cups young arugula leaves, rinsed and dried

- 1 cup cherry tomatoes, halved

- 1/4 cup pine nuts

- 2 tablespoons grapeseed oil or olive oil

- 1 tablespoon rice vinegar

- salt to taste

- freshly ground black pepper to taste

- 1/4 cup grated Parmesan cheese

- 1 large avocado—peeled, pitted and sliced

Instructions:

- In a large plastic bowl with a lid, combine arugula, cherry tomatoes, pine nuts, oil, vinegar, and Parmesan cheese. Season with salt and pepper to taste. Cover, and shake to mix.

Divide salad onto plates, and top with slices of avocado.

Cucumber Salad

Ingredients:

Original recipe makes 8 servings

- 3 cucumbers, seeded and sliced

- 1 1/2 cups crumbled feta cheese

- 1 cup black olives, pitted and sliced

- 3 cups diced roma tomatoes

- 1/3 cup diced oil packed sun-dried tomatoes, drained, oil reserved

- 1/2 red onion, sliced

- PREP 10 minutes

- **Instructions:**

In a large salad bowl, toss together the cucumbers, feta cheese, olives, roma tomatoes, sun-dried tomatoes, 2 tablespoons reserved sun-dried tomato oil, and red onion. Chill until serving.

SIDE DISHES

Sauteed Spinach with Pine Nuts & Golden Raisins

Makes: 2 servings Pine nuts and sweet golden raisins brighten up sauteed spinach.

Active Time: 15 minutes

Total Time: 15 minutes

Ingredients:

- 2 teaspoons extra-virgin olive oil

- 2 tablespoons golden raisins

- 1 tablespoon pine nuts

- 2 cloves garlic, minced

- 1 10-ounce bag fresh spinach

- 2 teaspoons balsamic vinegar

- 1/8 teaspoon salt

- 1 tablespoon shaved Parmesan cheese

- Freshly ground pepper, to taste

Instructions:

- Heat oil in a large nonstick skillet or Dutch oven over medium-high heat. Add raisins, pine nuts and garlic; cook, stirring, until fragrant, about 30 seconds. Add spinach and cook, stirring, until just wilted, about 2 minutes. Remove from heat; stir in vinegar and salt. Serve immediately, sprinkled with Parmesan and pepper.

Tips & Notes

- Note: The sturdier texture of mature spinach stands up better if you sauté than baby spinach and it's a more economical choice. We prefer to serve baby spinach raw.

Nutrition:

Per serving: 158 calories; 9 g fat (2 g sat, 5 g mono); 2 mg cholesterol; 16 g carbohydrates; 6 g protein; 4 g fiber; 310 mg sodium; 804 mg potassium.

Nutrition Bonus: Vitamin A (170% daily value), Folate (42% dv), Vitamin C (40% dv), Magnesium (29% dv), Potassium (23% dv), Calcium & Iron (20% dv)

Real Hummus

- *PREP 15 min*

READY IN 15 min

Ingredients :

Original recipe makes 2.5 cups

- 1 clove garlic

- 1 (19 ounce) can garbanzo beans, half the liquid reserved

- 4 tablespoons lemon juice

- 2 tablespoons tahini

- 1 clove garlic, chopped

- 1 teaspoon salt

- black pepper to taste

- 2 tablespoons olive oil

Instructions:

- In a blender, chop the garlic. Pour garbanzo beans into blender, reserving about a tablespoon for garnish. Place lemon juice, tahini, chopped garlic and salt in blender.

Blend until creamy and well mixed. Transfer the mixture to a medium-serving bowl. Sprinkle with pepper and pour olive oil over the top. Garnish with reserved garbanzo beans.

Mediterranean Kale

- *PREP 15 min*

- *COOK 10 min*

- *READY IN 25 min*

- **Ingredients:**

Original recipe makes 6 servings

- 12 cups chopped kale

- 2 tablespoons lemon juice

- 1 tablespoon olive oil, or as needed

- 1 tablespoon minced garlic

- 1 teaspoon soy sauce

- salt to taste

- ground black pepper to taste

- **Instructions:**

- Place a steamer insert into a saucepan, and fill with water to just below the bottom of the steamer. Cover, and bring the water to a boil over high heat. Add the kale, recover, and steam until just tender, 7 to 10 minutes depending on thickness. Whisk together the lemon juice, olive oil, garlic, soy sauce, salt, and black pepper in a large bowl. Toss steamed kale into dressing until well coated.

Roasted Eggplant & Feta Dip

Makes: 12 servings, about 1/4 cup each

Active Time: 40 minutes

Total Time: 40 minutes

From EatingWell

This roasted eggplant and feta dip gets a kick from a fresh Chile pepper and cayenne pepper. There are countless variations on this classic meze (appetizer) in Greece. Out-of-season eggplant or eggplant that has been heavily watered often has an abundance of seeds, which make the vegetable bitter. Be sure to taste the dip before you serve it; if it's a touch bitter, you can remedy that with a little sugar. Serve with toasted pita crisps or as a sandwich spread.

Ingredients:

- 1 medium eggplant (about 1 pound)

- 2 tablespoons lemon juice

- 1/4 cup extra-virgin olive oil

- 1/2 cup crumbled feta cheese, preferably Greek

- 1/2 cup finely chopped red onion

- 1 small red bell pepper, finely chopped

- 1 small Chile pepper, such as jalapeño, seeded and minced (optional)

- 2 tablespoons chopped fresh basil

- 1 tablespoon finely chopped flat-leaf parsley

- 1/4 teaspoon cayenne pepper, or to taste

- 1/4 teaspoon salt

- Pinch of sugar (optional)

- **Instructions:**

- Position oven rack about 6 inches from the heat source; preheat broiler. Line a baking pan with foil. Place eggplant in the pan and poke a few holes all over it to vent steam. Broil the eggplant, turning with tongs every 5 minutes, until the skin is charred and a knife inserted into the dense flesh near the stem goes in easily, 14 to 18 minutes. Transfer to a cutting board until cool enough to handle. Put lemon juice in a medium bowl. Cut the eggplant in half lengthwise and scrape the flesh into the bowl, tossing with the lemon juice to help prevent discoloring. Add oil and stir with a fork until the oil is absorbed. (It should be a little chunky.) Stir in feta, onion, bell pepper, Chile pepper (if using), basil, parsley, cayenne and salt. Taste and add sugar if needed.

Tips & Notes:

- Make Ahead Tip: Cover and refrigerate for up to 2 days.

Nutrition:

Per serving: 75 calories; 6 g fat (2 g sat, 4 g mono); 6 mg cholesterol; 4 g carbohydrates; 0 g added sugars; 2 g protein; 2 g fiber; 129 mg sodium; 121 mg potassium.

Lima Bean Spread with Cumin & Herbs From EatingWell

Humble lima beans are transformed into a sensational Mediterranean spread that is vibrant with a mix of fresh herbs and spices. You can substitute frozen edamame beans for the lima beans in Step 1; cook according to package directions.

Ingredients:

- 1 10-ounce package frozen lima beans

- 4 cloves garlic, crushed and peeled

- 1/4 teaspoon crushed red pepper

- 2 tablespoons extra-virgin olive oil

- 4 teaspoons lemon juice

- 1 teaspoon ground cumin

- 1/2 teaspoon salt, or to taste

- Freshly ground pepper, to taste

- 1 tablespoon chopped fresh mint

- 1 tablespoon chopped fresh cilantro

- 1 tablespoon chopped fresh dill

Instructions:

Bring a large saucepan of lightly salted water to a boil. Add lima beans, garlic and crushed red pepper; cook until the beans are tender, about 10 minutes. Remove from heat and let cool in the liquid. Drain the beans and garlic. Transfer to a food processor. Add oil, lemon juice, cumin, salt and pepper; process until smooth. Scrape into a bowl, stir in mint, cilantro and dill.

Tips & Notes

- Make Ahead Tip: Cover and refrigerate for up to 4 days or freeze for up to 6 months.

Nutrition:

Per tablespoon: 25 calories; 1 g fat (0 g sat, 1 g mono); 0 mg cholesterol; 3 g carbohydrates; 0 g added sugars; 1 g protein; 1 g fiber; 56 mg sodium; 62 mg potassium.

EGGPLANT WITH ALMONDS

PREP 40 min

COOK 35 min

READY IN 1 hr 35 min

Ingredients:

Original recipe makes 4 servings

- 2 large eggplants, cut into cubes

- salt

- 1/4 cup olive oil

- 1 large onion, minced

- 2 cloves garlic, minced

- 1 cup whole almonds, skin removed

- 2 cups cherry tomatoes, halved and seeded

- 4 mint leaves, sliced

- 2 tablespoons white wine

- 2 tablespoons white sugar

- 1 pinch salt

- 1/2 teaspoon chili powder

- 1/2 cup chopped fresh parsley

Instructions:

- Place the eggplant in a colander and sprinkle with salt. Set the colander in the sink to drain off liquid, about 20 minutes. Pat the cubes with paper towel to remove excess salt.

- Heat the olive oil in a large skillet over medium-high heat. Cook the onion in the oil until translucent. Add the garlic; cook and stir another 2 minutes. Stir in the eggplant and almonds, cooking and stirring until the eggplant is tender, but not mushy, about 20 minutes.

When the eggplant is cooked through, mix in the tomatoes, mint, white wine, sugar, salt, and chili powder. Cook mixture for 10 minutes, stirring occasionally; remove from heat and garnish with parsley.

Greek Zucchini

PREP 20 min

- *COOK 35 min*

- *READY IN 55 min*

Ingredients:

Original recipe makes 4 servings

- 1 medium zucchini, halved and sliced

- 1/4 cup diced red onion

- 1/4 cup diced green bell pepper

- 2 (4 ounce) cans sliced black olives, drained

- 1/4 cup crumbled feta cheese

- 2 tablespoons Greek vinaigrette salad dressing

- 1/4 cup grape or cherry tomatoes, halved

Instructions:

- Preheat oven to 350 degrees F (175 degrees C). Spray a large piece of aluminum foil with nonstick cooking spray. Layer the zucchini, onion, pepper, and olives onto the center.

Sprinkle with feta cheese, and drizzle with vinaigrette. Fold into a packet and seal the edges. Bake in preheated oven until vegetables are tender, about 30 minutes. Open the foil packet, turn the oven onto Broil, and broil until the feta lightly browns. Add the grape tomatoes and serve.

OLIVE AND EGGPLANT DIP

Briny olives bring a gratifying richness to this Mediterranean-inspired eggplant dip.

Ingredients:

- 2 Italian eggplants (10 ounces each), halved lengthwise

- 1 1/2 teaspoons extra-virgin olive oil

- 1 garlic clove, thinly sliced

- 1/4 teaspoon coarse salt

- 1/2 cup pitted Kalamata olives

- 1/2 cup pitted green olives, such as Picholine or Sicilian

- 1 teaspoon finely chopped fresh oregano, plus small leaves for garnish

- 1 teaspoon finely grated lemon zest, plus long strips zest for garnish

- Pinch of red-pepper flakes

- 2 yellow bell peppers, seeds and ribs removed, flesh cut into 1 1/2-inch pieces

Instructions:

- Preheat oven to 400 degrees. Place eggplants cut sides up, on a rimmed baking sheet, and brush with 1/2-teaspoon oil. Scatter garlic over tops, and sprinkle with salt. Roast until golden and tender, about 20 minutes. Let cool slightly.

- Remove eggplant seeds- spoon flesh and garlic into a food processor. Puree; transfer to a medium bowl.

Add olives to processor, and pulse until coarsely chopped. Add to bowl with eggplant mixture. Stir in chopped oregano, lemon zest, red-pepper flakes, and remaining teaspoon oil. Garnish with oregano leaves and lemon-zest strips. Serve with bell peppers.

Golden Bruschetta

- *Yield Serves 4*

- You can simplify this bruschetta even more by grilling, drizzling very good quality olive oil, and lightly salting the bread

- **Ingredients**

- Four 1/4-inch-thick slices brioche

- 1/2 pound pear tomatoes, halved

- 1/2 cup assorted fresh herbs (basil, tarragon, thyme, dill, chives)

- 2 teaspoons extra-virgin olive oil

- Kosher salt and freshly ground black pepper

Instructions:

- Grill or toast the bread slices until golden and crisp. Set aside. In a small bowl, toss together the tomatoes, herbs, olive oil, and salt and pepper. Spoon a quarter of the mixture onto each brioche slice, season with additional pepper, and serve.

Warm Olives

Ingredients:

- 4 ounces green olives

- 4 ounces black olives

- 1/4 cup olive oil

- 1 sprig rosemary

- 1/4 teaspoon fennel seeds

- 1 pinch crushed red pepper

Instructions:

Heat all ingredients in a skillet over medium. Sauté, tossing until starting to brown (3 minutes). Serve warm or at room temperature.

Mediterranean Stuffed Tomatoes

Ingredients:

- 2 large tomatoes

- 1/2 cup packaged garlic croutons

- 1/4 cup (1 ounce) crumbled goat cheese

- 1/4 cup sliced pitted kalamata olives

- 2 tablespoons reduced-fat vinaigrette or Italian salad dressing

- 2 tablespoons chopped fresh thyme or basil

Instructions:

Preheat broiler. Cut tomatoes in half crosswise. Use your finger to push out and discard seeds; use a paring knife to cut out the pulp, leaving 2 shells. Chop pulp, and transfer to a medium bowl. Place hollowed tomatoes, cut sides down, on a paper towel; drain 5 minutes. Add croutons, goat cheese, olives, dressing, and thyme or basil to pulp; mix well. Mound mixture into hollowed tomatoes. Place tomatoes on a baking sheet or broiler pan. Broil 4-5 inches from heat until hot and cheese melts (about 5 minutes). Serve immediately.

MAIN DISHES

Turkey-Hummus Sliders

Ingredients:

1 cucumber, diced

1/2 cup crumbled feta cheese

2 tablespoons red wine vinegar

1 teaspoon dried mint

4 tablespoons extra-virgin olive oil

Kosher salt and freshly ground pepper

1 1/2 pounds ground turkey

1 cup hummus, preferably spicy or roasted red pepper (about a 7-ounce container)

1/2 cup chopped fresh parsley

2 teaspoons ground coriander

16 mini pita pockets, preferably whole wheat, split open and warmed

2 to 3 plum tomatoes, sliced

Instructions:

Toss the cucumber, feta, vinegar, mint, 1 tablespoon olive oil and a pinch each of salt and pepper in a bowl; cover and refrigerate. Mix the turkey, 1/2 cup hummus, the parsley and coriander in a bowl; season generously with pepper. Dampen your hands and shape the mixture into 16 small patties, about 1/2 inch thick.Heat 1 1/2 tablespoons olive oil in a medium cast-iron skillet over medium-high heat. Add half of the patties and cook until browned and cooked through, about 2 minutes per side. Transfer to a plate. Cook the remaining patties in the remaining 1 1/2 tablespoons olive oil. Mix the remaining 1/2 cup hummus with a splash of hot water in a bowl. Spread some of the hummus on the inside of each pita; fill with a tomato slice, turkey patty and some of the cucumber mixture.

Cube Steak Milanese

Makes: 4 servings, 1 steak & 1 1/2 cups salad each

Active Time: 45 minutes

Total Time: 45 minutes

From Eating Well: The economical cube steak is elevated to new heights in this recipe. The salad, with chopped arugula, basil, tomatoes, onion and sharp Italian cheese, is the picture of summer simplicity; all it needs is olive oil and lemon to dress it.

Ingredients:

- 4 plum tomatoes, seeded and chopped
- 1/2 cup diced red onion
- 1/2 teaspoon salt, divided
- 1 egg, plus 1 egg white
- 1/2 cup plain dry breadcrumbs
- 1/4 cup grated Pecorino Romano, or Parmesan cheese plus 1/4 cup shaved (see Tip), divided
- 2 tablespoons minced fresh parsley,
- 1 pound cube steak, cut into 4 portions
- 1/2 teaspoon freshly ground pepper, divided
- 6 teaspoons extra-virgin olive oil, divided
- 4 cups baby arugula, chopped
- 3/4 cup thinly sliced fresh basil leaves
- 1 tablespoon fresh lemon juice, plus lemon wedges for garnish

- **Instructions:**

Combine tomatoes, onion and 1/4 teaspoon salt in a large bowl. Whisk egg and egg white in a shallow dish. Combine breadcrumbs, grated cheese and parsley (if using) in another shallow dish. Season steak with the remaining 1/4 teaspoon salt and 1/4 teaspoon pepper. Dip each piece into the egg, allowing excess to drip off into the dish, then dip in the breadcrumb mixture and turn to coat.

Heat 2 teaspoons oil in a large nonstick skillet over medium heat. Add the steaks and cook until golden brown on the first side, about 3 minutes. Turn the steaks over, add 1 teaspoon oil and cook until the steaks are cooked through, 3 to 4 minutes more. Transfer to a plate; tent with foil to keep warm.

Add 1/4 cup shaved cheese to the tomato mixture. Add the remaining 1/4 teaspoon pepper, the remaining 3 teaspoons oil, arugula, basil and lemon juice; toss to combine. Serve the steaks on beds of the arugula-tomato salad. Garnish with lemon wedges.

- **Tips:**

- Tip: Use a vegetable peeler to shave hard Italian cheese, such as Parmesan or Pecorino Romano.

Nutrition:

Per serving: 348 calories; 17 g fat (5 g sat, 6 g mono); 130 mg cholesterol; 14 g carbohydrates; 35 g protein; 2 g fiber; 581 mg sodium; 339 mg potassium.

Nutrition Bonus: Vitamin A (30% daily value), Vitamin C & Iron (25% dv), Folate (16% dv),

Chicken, Broccoli Rabe & Feta on Toast

From Eating Well: The assertive flavor of broccoli rabe can be a schoolyard bully in dishes. But here, the sweet tomatoes and briny feta stand up to its bite, rendering this dish a rustic but comforting favorite. Still, if broccoli rabe proves too strong for your taste, you can substitute broccolini or even tiny, trimmed broccoli florets.

Ingredients:

- 4 thick slices whole-wheat country bread

- 1 clove garlic, peeled (optional), plus 1/4 cup chopped garlic

- 4 teaspoons extra-virgin olive oil, divided

- 1 pound chicken tenders, cut crosswise into 1/2-inch pieces

- 1 bunch broccoli rabe, stems trimmed, cut into 1-inch pieces, or 2 bunches broccolini, chopped (see Ingredient note)

- 2 cups cherry tomatoes, halved

- 1 tablespoon red-wine vinegar

- 1/8 teaspoon salt

- Freshly ground pepper, to taste

- 3/4 cup crumbled feta cheese

Instructions:

- Grill or toast bread. Lightly rub with peeled garlic clove, if desired. Discard the garlic.

- Heat 2 teaspoons oil in a large nonstick skillet over high heat until shimmering but not smoking. Add chicken; cook, stirring occasionally, until just cooked through and no longer pink in the middle, 4 to 5 minutes. Transfer the chicken and any juices to a plate; cover to keep warm.

- Add the remaining 2 teaspoons oil to the pan. Add chopped garlic and cook, stirring constantly, until fragrant but not brown, about 30 seconds. Add broccoli rabe (or broccolini) and cook, stirring often, until bright green and just wilted, 2 to 4 minutes. Stir in tomatoes, vinegar, salt and pepper; cook, stirring occasionally, until the tomatoes are beginning to break down, 2 to 4 minutes. Return the chicken and juices to the pan, add feta cheese and stir to combine. Cook until heated through, 1 to 2 minutes. Serve warm over garlic toasts.

- **Tips and Notes:**

- Ingredient Note: Pleasantly pungent and mildly bitter, broccoli rabe, or rapini, is a member of the cabbage family and commonly used in Mediterranean cooking. Broccolini (a cross between broccoli and Chinese kale) is sweet and tender—the florets and stalks are edible.

Nutrition:

Per serving: 313 calories; 11 g fat (5 g sat, 5 g mono); 85 mg cholesterol; 26 g carbohydrates; 35 g protein; 4 g fiber; 653 mg sodium; 423 mg potassium.

Nutrition Bonus: Vitamin C (160% daily value), Vitamin A (140% dv), Selenium (28% dv),

Curry Rubbed Salmon with Napa Slaw

Broiling makes the salmon golden brown without adding fat. To get the best color and a crisp coat, don't turn the fish over while cooking; it will still cook all the way through without this extra step.

Nutrition: Per serving: 597 calories; 45 g protein; 20 g fat; 57 g carb; 6 g fiber

Ingredients:

1 cup brown basmati rice

- Coarse salt and ground pepper

- 1 pound Napa cabbage (1/2 head), thinly sliced crosswise

- 1 pound carrots, coarsely grated

- 1/2 cup fresh mint leaves

- 1/4 cup fresh lime juice, plus lime wedges for serving

- 2 tablespoons grapeseed oil

- 4 salmon filets (6 ounces each)

- 2 teaspoons curry powder

Instructions:

- In a large saucepan, bring 2 cups water to a boil; add rice. Season with salt and pepper, cover, and reduce heat to medium-low. Cook until tender, 30 to 35 minutes.

- Meanwhile, in a large bowl, combine cabbage, carrots, mint, lime juice, and oil; season with salt and pepper. Toss.

Heat broiler with rack set 4 inches from heat. About 10 minutes before rice is done cooking, place salmon on a foil-lined rimmed baking sheet. Rub salmon with curry, and season with salt and pepper. Broil until just cooked through, 6 to 8 minutes. Fluff rice with a fork and serve alongside salad and salmon.

Whole-Wheat Greek Pizza

There's no need to buy a special pizza pan; an upside-down baking sheet works just as well. If you like, you can add a little cornmeal to the baking sheet before cooking.

- *Prep Time 10 minutes*

- *Total Time 30 minutes*

- *Yield Serves 4*

Ingredients:

- 2 tablespoons olive oil, plus more for baking sheet

- 1 cup cherry tomatoes

- 1 clove garlic, coarsely chopped

- Coarse salt and freshly ground pepper

- Whole-wheat flour, for work surface

- 1 pound whole-wheat pizza dough,

- 1 cup (4 ounces) grated haloumi cheese

- 2 tablespoons pine nuts

- 2 cups baby arugula

- 1 tablespoon red-wine vinegar

- 1/4 cup pitted kalamata olives, coarsely chopped

Instructions:

- Preheat oven to 450 degrees. Turn a large baking sheet upside down; rub with oil. Place tomatoes, garlic, and 1 tablespoon oil in a food processor; season with salt and pepper. Pulse 3 to 4 times until ingredients are incorporated but chunky.

- On a lightly floured work surface, use a rolling pin and your hands to roll and stretch dough until large enough to cover the surface of the baking sheet. (If dough becomes too elastic, let it rest a few minutes.) Transfer to prepared baking sheet.

- Spread tomato sauce evenly over dough, leaving a 1-inch border all around. Top with cheese and pine nuts; season with salt and pepper.

Bake until crust is golden, 15 to 20 minutes. Toss arugula with vinegar and 1 tablespoon oil; season with salt and pepper. Sprinkle arugula and olives over pizza.

Zucchini Pie

Marjoram, with its hint of balsam, complements mild yellow and green summer squash in this simple crustless zucchini pie. It is topped by tomato slices and low-fat feta cheese, a lean choice. If yellow zucchini are unavailable, use all green zucchini.

Ingredients:

- 2 teaspoons olive oil

- 1 pound (about 2 or 3) green zucchini, cut into 1/2-inch pieces

- 4 scallions, thinly sliced

- 4 cloves garlic, minced

- 1 teaspoon dried marjoram

- 1 teaspoon coarse salt

- 1/2 teaspoon freshly ground pepper

- 1 pound (about 2 or 3) yellow zucchini, cut into 1/2-inch pieces

- 1/2 cup freshly chopped dill

- 1/4 cup freshly chopped flat-leaf parsley

- 5 large eggs plus 5 large egg whites, lightly beaten

- 1 tomato, thinly sliced

- 2 ounces low-fat feta cheese, crumbled

Instructions:

Preheat oven to 325 degrees. Heat 1 teaspoon olive oil in a large skillet set over medium heat. Add green zucchini, half the scallions, half the garlic, A teaspoon marjoram, 1/2 teaspoon salt, and 1/4 teaspoon pepper; cook, stirring frequently, until zucchini has softened and is beginning to brown, about 5 minutes. Remove from heat; transfer to a large bowl; set aside.

Rinse skillet; repeat process with yellow zucchini and remaining teaspoon olive oil, scallions, garlic, 1/2 teaspoon marjoram, 1/2 teaspoon salt, and 1/4 teaspoon pepper. Transfer to bowl with cooked green zucchini; let sit until cooled. Drain and discard any liquid.

Add dill, parsley, and eggs to zucchini; stir to combine. Pour into a 9 1/2-inch round, deep baking dish. Cover with tomato; sprinkle with feta. Bake until set, about 1 hour. Serve hot or at room temperature.

Moussaka

Eggplant is layered with a mixture of low-fat turkey, tomatoes, onions, garlic, and spices and topped with a light yogurt sauce in our version of moussaka, a Mediterranean classic. Moussaka may be assembled a day in advance and refrigerated; bake for an additional 15 to 20 minutes or until center is hot.

Ingredients:

- 2 cups plain nonfat yogurt

- 1 pound ground turkey

- 1 yellow onion, cut into 1/4-inch dice

- 1 clove garlic, minced

- 1 teaspoon ground cinnamon

- 1 teaspoon coarse salt, plus more for eggplant

- 1/4 teaspoon ground nutmeg

- 1/4 teaspoon freshly ground pepper

- One 28-ounce can whole peeled tomatoes, coarsely chopped

- 1/4 cup tomato paste

- 1/4 cup chopped fresh oregano

- 1/2 cup chopped fresh flat-leaf parsley

- 2 medium eggplants (about 2 pounds)

- 1/4 cup (1 ounce) grated Parmesan cheese

- 1 large egg, plus 1 large egg white

- Olive-oil, cooking spray

Instructions:

Drain yogurt in a cheesecloth-lined sieve until thickened, 2 hours or overnight.

Place turkey in a medium saucepan over medium heat; cook until browned, about 6 minutes. Using a slotted spoon, transfer to a medium bowl. Add onion, garlic, cinnamon, salt, nutmeg, and pepper to saucepan; cook until onion is translucent, about 10 minutes. Return turkey to saucepan with tomatoes, tomato paste, and oregano. Bring to a boil; reduce heat to medium low; simmer until sauce has thickened, about 1 hour. Remove from heat; stir in chopped parsley; set aside.

Preheat broiler. While sauce cooks, cut eggplants into 1/4-inch slices. Sprinkle with salt on both sides. Place in a colander over a bowl; let stand 1 hour to drain. Discard liquid; rinse each slice under cold running water to remove all salt and juice. Place slices on several layers of paper towels; press out water. Lay dry slices on a clean baking sheet; coat with olive-oil spray; broil until browned, about 2 minutes. Turn; coat with olive-oil spray; broil until browned, about 2 minutes more. Repeat until all eggplant slices have been broiled; set cooked eggplant aside.

Place drained yogurt in a small bowl. Add Parmesan and eggs. Whisk together briskly with a fork; set aside.

Preheat oven to 400 degrees. Assemble moussaka: Place a layer of eggplant on the bottom of an 8-by-8-inch baking pan. Cover with half the turkey sauce. Place another eggplant layer, then the remaining turkey sauce. Add a final eggplant layer; cover with reserved yogurt mixture. Bake until mixture is bubbling and top starts to brown, about 30 minutes. Transfer to a heat-proof surface;

let sit until moussaka cools slightly and firms, about 10 minutes. Cut into squares; serve.

Mediterranean Chicken Wrap

Chicken provides a great source of protein, while the tapenade adds healthy fats. Artichoke hearts and tomato bring fiber to the table. The whole-wheat wrap offers a better carb choice than a white wrap.

Adapted Body+Soul

- *Prep Time 10 minutes*

- *Total Time 10 minutes*

- *Yield Serves 1*

Ingredients:

- 1 chicken breast

- Coarse salt and ground pepper

- 1 whole-wheat wrap, 10 inches

- 1 tablespoon olive tapenade

- 2 cans artichoke hearts, squeezed dry and thinly sliced

- 1/2 small tomato, thinly sliced

- 1/4 cup mixed baby greens

Instructions:

Cook chicken (or grabbed grilled chicken already made). Spread bottom of wrap with the olive tapenade. Layer with chicken, artichoke hearts, tomato, and baby greens; season with salt and pepper. Fold tortilla to seal.

Mediterranean Pasta with Artichokes and Olives

Whole-wheat pasta has almost twice the amount of fiber of traditional semolina pasta.

Body+Soul

Prep Time 15 minutes

- *Total Time 25 minutes*

- *Yield Serves 4*

Ingredients:

- Coarse salt and ground pepper

- 12 ounces whole-wheat spaghetti

- 2 tablespoons olive oil

- 1/2 medium onion, thinly sliced, lengthwise

- 2 garlic cloves, thinly sliced crosswise

- 1/2 cup dry white wine

- 1/2 cup fresh basil leaves, torn

- 1 can artichoke hearts, drained, rinsed, and quartered lengthwise

- 1/3 cup pitted kalamata olives, quartered lengthwise

- 1 pint cherry or grape tomatoes, halved lengthwise

- 1/4 cup grated Parmesan cheese, plus more serving

Instructions:

- In a large pot of boiling salted water, cook pasta until al dente according to package directions. Drain, reserving 1 cup of pasta water. Return pasta to pot.

- Meanwhile, in a large skillet, heat 1 tablespoon oil over medium-high. Add onion and garlic, season with salt and pepper, cook, stirring occasionally until browned, 3 to 4 minutes. Add wine and cook until evaporated, about 2 minutes.

Stir in artichokes and cook until starting to brown, 2 to 3 minutes. Add olives and half of the tomatoes; cook until tomatoes start to break down, 1 to 2 minutes. Add pasta to skillet. Stir in remaining tomatoes, oil, cheese, and basil. Thin with reserved pasta water if necessary to coat the spaghetti. Serve with additional cheese.

Ginger Shrimp with Charred Tomato Relish

- Green tomatoes are simply unripe red tomatoes — hence their lower sugar content and slightly sour taste. Charring makes them softer and easier to peel. To grill the shrimp use 8-inch wooden skewers, which you'll find in some supermarkets and kitchenware stores.

Body+Soul

- *Prep Time 45 minutes*

- *Total Time 1 hour 20 minutes*

- *Yield Serves 4*

Ingredients:

- 2 garlic cloves, minced

- 1 1/2 tablespoons grated peeled ginger (2-inch piece)

- 3 tablespoons vegetable oil, plus more for grill

- 20 extra-large shrimp (about 1 pound), peeled, deveined, tails left on

- 4 ripe plum tomatoes, halved lengthwise

- 2 medium green tomatoes, halved lengthwise

- Coarse salt and freshly ground black pepper

- 2 tablespoons fresh lime juice (1 lime)

- 1 tablespoon minced fresh jalapeno pepper (with seeds)

- 1 teaspoon sugar

- 1 tablespoon chopped cilantro

- 1 tablespoon chopped basil

Instructions:

- Soak 20 skewers in a pan of water for 30 minutes.

- In a medium bowl, stir together garlic and ginger. Transfer half of the mixture to a large bowl and stir in 2 tablespoons oil. Add the shrimp, toss until evenly coated, and then cover and refrigerate for 30 minutes. Cover remaining garlic-ginger mixture and refrigerate.

- Heat grill to hot; lightly oil grates. In a medium bowl toss plum and green tomatoes with remaining tablespoon oil; season with salt and pepper. Grill tomatoes, cut side up, until skins are charred and flesh is tender, 4 to 6 minutes for the plum tomatoes, 8 to 10 minutes for the green tomatoes (if the green tomatoes are very hard, this may take longer). Be careful as you grill, as the juice from the tomatoes and the oil on their surface may cause flare-ups.

- When tomatoes are cool enough to handle, remove and discard skins and seeds. Finely chop flesh and add to bowl with reserved garlic-ginger mixture. Add lime juice, jalapeno, sugar, cilantro, and basil.

- Season shrimp with salt and pepper. Thread shrimp, lengthwise, onto prepared skewers (going through tail and top of shrimp), one shrimp per skewer. Grill until shrimp are opaque throughout, about 2 minutes per side.

To serve, place skewered shrimp on a platter with a bowl of the relish.

Garlic-Braised Chicken with Olives and Mushrooms

When it's no longer winter but not quite spring, a savory stovetop braise, served over rustic grains like faro. Makes a comforting weeknight meal. Braised garlic is a sweet counterpart to briny olives, earthy mushrooms, and succulent chicken. Simmering it all in stock will enrich the flavors.

Body+Soul

- Yield Serves 4

Ingredients:

- 1 small chicken (about 2 1/2 pounds), cut into pieces

- Coarse salt and freshly ground pepper

- 1 tablespoon plus 1 teaspoon olive oil

- 2 heads garlic (at least 16 cloves), smashed and peeled

- 10 ounces mushrooms, cleaned, trimmed, and halved

- 1/2 cup white wine

- , 1/2 cup green olives pitted or left whole

- 1/3 cup chicken stock

Instructions:

- Heat a large straight-sided skillet (about 12 inches) over medium-high heat. While it's heating, season chicken with salt and pepper. Add 1 tablespoon oil to pan and swirl. Add chicken, skin side down. Let brown, 5 to 6 minutes. Remove chicken from pan; set aside.

- Add 1 teaspoon oil to pan, followed by garlic and mushrooms; let brown, stirring occasionally, 5 to 6 minutes.

- Add wine to mushrooms and garlic and bring to a boil, then cook for 1 minute. Return chicken to pan.

Add olives and chicken stock to pan; bring to a boil, then reduce heat. Cover; simmer until chicken is cooked through, 15 to 20 minutes.

Linguine with Two-Olive Tapenade

- Yield Serves 4

Tapenade made with two types of olives, garlic, parsley, and lemon zest makes a delectable sauce for linguine. Chunks of tuna and cherry tomatoes complete the dish. Serve it with a salad for a light meal. The tapenade can also be served as a dip for crudites or a zesty sauce for grilled fish. For best results, choose olives with distinctive flavors, such as those suggested below.

Martha Stewart Living

Ingredients:

- 1/2 pound linguine

- One 6-ounce can tuna, packed in water, drained

- 1 1/2 cups cherry tomatoes, quartered

For The Tapenade

1/3 cup pitted brine-cured olives, such as Kalamata (about 16)

1/3 cup pitted ripe green olives, such as Picholine (about 18)

Finely grated zest of 1 lemon

2 garlic cloves

2 tablespoons plus 1/3 cup roughly chopped fresh flat-leaf parsley, plus whole sprigs for garnish

1/2 teaspoon freshly ground black pepper

1/4 teaspoon crushed red-pepper flakes

Instructions:

- Bring a large pot of water to a boil. Add linguine; cook according to package instructions, stirring occasionally, until it is al dente. Remove from heat, and transfer linguine to a colander; let drain, reserving 1/4 cup cooking water.

- Make tapenade: In the bowl of a food processor fitted with the metal blade, combine olives, lemon zest, garlic, 2 tablespoons parsley, black pepper, and red-pepper flakes. Process until mixture is finely chopped and combined.

Transfer linguine to a large serving bowl, and toss with reserved cooking water. Add tapenade, tuna, tomatoes, and remaining 1/3 cup chopped parsley; toss well to coat. Serve immediately, garnished with parsley sprigs.

Mediterranean Seafood Grill with Skordalia

Ingredients:

- 1 pound russet or Yukon gold potatoes

- 8 garlic cloves, peeled

- 1 slice sourdough bread, crust removed

- 1/4 cup plain Greek low-fat yogurt

- 3 tablespoons olive oil, divided

- Zest and juice of 1 lemon

- 1/2 teaspoon salt, divided

- 1/4 teaspoon dried thyme

- 1 pound halibut fillets, cut into 4 pieces

- 2 red bell peppers, quartered

- 1 pound small zucchini, diagonally cut into 1-inch pieces

- 1/2 red onion, sliced

Instructions:

Peel potatoes, and chop into 1-inch pieces. Place in a large saucepan, and cover with cold water. Add garlic, and cook over high heat about 15 minutes or until potatoes are easily pierced with a fork.

While potatoes cook, tear bread into 3 or 4 pieces and place in a large bowl. Spoon 2 to 3 tablespoons cooking liquid from potatoes over bread. Stir with a fork until smooth. Add yogurt, 2 tablespoons olive oil, and zest and juice of 1 lemon; stir until a smooth paste forms.

When the potatoes are done, place a large bowl in the sink and set a colander on top. Drain potatoes and garlic, reserving cooking liquid. Transfer potatoes to bread mixture and mash until smooth (a potato ricer works well for this task). Add reserved cooking liquid 2 tablespoons at a time until mixture takes on the consistency of loose mashed potatoes. Stir in ï¿½ teaspoon salt and 2 teaspoons olive oil. Cover and keep warm until ready to serve.

Preheat grill pan over medium-high heat. Drizzle fish with ï¿½ teaspoon olive oil and season with remaining ï¿½ teaspoon salt and thyme. Cook fish 2 to 3 minutes on each side until fish flakes when tested with a fork or until desired degree of doneness. Transfer to a plate; cover and keep warm until ready to serve.

5 Place bell pepper, zucchini, and red onion in a large bowl. Drizzle with remaining ï¿½ teaspoon olive oil; toss to coat. Arrange bell pepper in grill pan and cook 5 minutes over medium heat. Add zucchini and onion; cook 10 minutes or until vegetables are tender, turning as necessary to ensure even cooking.

Calories per serving:	390
Fat per serving:	14g

Mediterranean Chickpea Patties

Ingredients:

- 1 (15.5-ounce) can chickpeas, rinsed and drained

- 1/2 cup fresh flat-leaf parsley

- 1 garlic clove, chopped

- 1/4 teaspoon ground cumin

- 1/2 teaspoon kosher salt, divided

- 1/2 teaspoon black pepper, divided

- 1 egg, whisked

- 4 tablespoons all-purpose flour, divided

- 2 tablespoons olive oil

- 1/2 cup low-fat Greek-style yogurt

- 3 tablespoons fresh lemon juice

- 8 cups mixed salad greens

- 1 cup grape tomatoes, halved

- 1/2 small red onion, thinly sliced

Pita chips (optional)

Instructions:

Pulse first 4 ingredients (through cumin) and 1/4 teaspoon each salt and pepper in a food processor until coarsely chopped and mixture comes together. Transfer to a bowl, add egg and 2 tablespoons flour; form into 8 (1/2-inch-thick) patties. Place remaining flour in a small dish and roll patties in it with floured hands; tap off excess flour. Heat oil in a nonstick skillet over medium-high heat. Cook patties for 2-3 minutes per side or until golden. Whisk together the yogurt, lemon juice, and remaining salt and pepper. Divide greens, tomatoes, onion, and patties evenly among 4 plates; drizzle each salad with 2 tablespoons dressing. Serve with pita chips, if desired.

Calories per serving:	225
Fat per serving:	8g

Mediterranean Salmon

Ingredients:

- 1/4 teaspoon salt

- 1/4 teaspoon black pepper

- 4 (6-ounce) skinless salmon fillets (about 1 inch thick)

- Cooking spray

- 2 cups cherry tomatoes, halved

- 1/2 cup finely chopped zucchini

- 2 tablespoons capers, undrained

- 1 tablespoon olive oil

- 1 (2 1/4-ounce) can sliced ripe olives, drained

Instructions:

Preheat oven to 425°. Sprinkle salt and pepper over both sides of fish. Place fish in a single layer in an 11- x 7-inch baking dish coated with cooking spray. Combine tomatoes and remaining ingredients in a bowl; spoon mixture over fish. Bake at 425° for 22 minutes.

Calories per serving:	339

Salmon Burgers

Ingredients:

- 1 pound skinless salmon fillets, cut into 2-inch pieces

- 1/2 cup panko

- 1 large egg white

- 1 pinch kosher salt

- 1/4 teaspoon freshly ground black pepper

- 1/2 cup cucumber slices

- 1/4 cup crumbled feta cheese

- 4 (2.5-oz) ciabatta rolls, toasted

Instructions:

In the bowl of a food processor, pulse salmon, panko, and egg white until salmon is finely chopped. Form salmon into 4 (4-inch) patties; season with salt and pepper. Heat grill to medium-high; cook, turning once, until burgers are just cooked through (5-7 minutes per side). Serve with desired toppings and buns.

Vegetable and Garlic Calzone

Ingredients:

- 3 asparagus stalks, cut into 1-inch pieces

- 1/2 cup chopped spinach

- 1/2 cup chopped broccoli

- 1/2 cup sliced mushrooms

- 2 tablespoons garlic, minced

- 2 teaspoons olive oil

- 1/2 pound frozen whole-wheat bread dough loaf, thawed

- 1 medium tomato, sliced

- 1/2 cup mozzarella cheese, shredded

- 2/3 cup pizza sauce

Instructions:

Preheat the oven to 400 F. Lightly coat a baking sheet with cooking spray.

In a medium bowl, add the asparagus, spinach, broccoli, mushrooms and garlic. Drizzle 1 teaspoon of the olive oil over the vegetables and toss to mix well.

Heat a large, nonstick frying pan over medium-high heat. Add the vegetables and saute for 4 to 5 minutes, stirring frequently. Remove from heat and set aside to cool.

On a floured surface, cut the bread dough in half. Press each half into a circle. Using a rolling pin, roll the dough into an oval.

On half of the oval, add 1/2 of the sauteed vegetables, 1/2 of the tomato slices and 1/4 cup cheese. Wet your finger and rub the edge of the dough that has the filling on it. Fold the dough over the filling, pressing the edges together. Roll the edges and then press them down with a fork. Place the calzone on the prepared baking sheet. Repeat to make the other calzone.Brush the calzones with the remaining 1 teaspoon olive oil. Bake until golden brown, about 20 minutes.Heat the pizza sauce in the microwave or on the stove top. Place each calzone on a plate. Serve with 1/3 cup pizza sauce on the side or pour the sauce over the calzones.

Nutritional analysis per serving

Serving size :1 calzone

Calories: 290

Grilled Salmon

Ingredients:

- 4 tablespoons chopped fresh basil

- 1 tablespoon chopped fresh parsley

- 1 tablespoon minced garlic

- 2 tablespoons lemon juice

- 4 salmon fillets, each 5 ounces

- Cracked black pepper, to taste

- 4 green olives, chopped

- 4 thin slices lemon

Instructions:

Prepare a hot fire in a charcoal grill or heat a gas grill or broiler. Away from the heat source, lightly coat the grill rack or broiler pan with cooking spray. Position the cooking rack 4 to 6 inches from the heat source. In a small bowl, combine the basil, parsley, minced garlic and lemon juice. Spray the fish with cooking spray. Sprinkle with black pepper. Top each fillet with equal amounts of the basil-garlic mixture. Place the fish herb-side down on the grill. Grill over high heat. When the edges turn white, after about 3 to 4 minutes, turn the fish over and place on aluminum foil. Move the fish to a cooler part of the grill or reduce the heat. Grill until the fish is opaque throughout when tested with the tip of a knife and an instant-read thermometer inserted into the thickest part of the fish reads 145 F (about 4 minutes longer). Remove the salmon and place on warmed plates. Garnish with green olives and lemon slices.

Nutritional analysis per serving

Serving size :1 fillet Calories 183

Mediterranean Shrimp and Pasta

Ingredients:

2 teaspoons olive oil

- Cooking spray

- 2 garlic cloves, minced

- 1 pound medium shrimp, peeled and deveined

- 2 cups chopped plum tomato

- 1/4 cup thinly sliced fresh basil

- 1/3 cup chopped pitted kalamata olives

- 2 tablespoons capers, drained

- 1/4 teaspoon freshly ground black pepper

- 4 cups hot cooked angel hair pasta (about 8 ounces uncooked pasta)

- 1/4 cup (2 ounces) crumbled feta cheese

Instructions:

Heat olive oil in a large nonstick skillet coated with cooking spray over medium-high heat. Add garlic; sauté 30 seconds. Add shrimp; sauté 1 minute. Add tomato and basil; reduce heat, and simmer 3 minutes or until tomato is tender. Stir in kalamata olives, capers, and black pepper.

Combine shrimp mixture and pasta in a large bowl; toss well. Top with cheese.

end of ingredients-prep

GREEK CHICKEN PASTA

PREP 15 mins

COOK 15 mins

READY IN 30 mins

Original recipe makes 6 servings

- **Ingredients:**

- 1 (16 ounce) package whole-wheat linguine pasta

- 1/2 cup chopped red onion

- 1 tablespoon olive oil

- 2 cloves garlic, crushed

- 1 pound skinless, boneless chicken breast meat–cut into bite-size pieces

- 1 (14 ounce) can marinated artichoke hearts, drained and chopped

- 1 large tomato, chopped

- 1/2 cup crumbled feta cheese

- 3 tablespoons chopped fresh parsley

- 2 tablespoons lemon juice

- 2 teaspoons dried oregano

- salt and pepper to taste

- 2 lemons, wedged, for garnish

Instructions:

- Bring a large pot of lightly salted water to a boil. Cook pasta in boiling water until tender yet firm to the bit, 8 to 10 minutes; drain.

- Heat olive oil in a large skillet over medium-high heat. Add onion and garlic; saute until fragrant, about 2 minutes. Stir in the chicken and cook, stirring occasionally, until chicken is no longer pink in the center and the juices run clear, about 5 to 6 minutes.

Reduce heat to medium-low; add artichoke hearts, tomato, feta cheese, parsley, lemon juice, oregano, and cooked pasta. Cook and stir until heated through, about 2 to 3 minutes. Remove from heat, season with salt and pepper, and garnish with lemon wedges.

DESSERTS

Mediterranean Style Baked Apple

Ingredients:

- 4 cooking apples (Granny Smiths or your favorite cooking apple)

- 4 tablespoons honey

- 1/2 teaspoon ground cinnamon

- ¼ teaspoon nutmeg

- ¼ teaspoon allspice

- 1/2 cup chopped walnuts or almonds

- 1/2 cup chopped golden raisins

- Juice of ½ lemon

- Lemon zest from ½ lemon

Instructions:

- Preheat oven to 350 degrees Fahrenheit. Core apples. Place the apples into a baking dish. Mix all other ingredients together. Fill the center core holes with the mixture making sure to push it firmly into the holes. Use the remaining filling mixture to form mounds on the top of the apples. Pour approximately ½ inch of water into the baking dish. Place on the middle shelf of the preheated oven. Bake at 350 degrees Fahrenheit approximately 40–45 minutes (the apple will be soft).Place apples on serving plates. Pour the juices from the baking dish over the apples. Serve immediately.

Fruit Salad with Honey Mint Sauce

Ingredients:

- ¼ cup strawberries, quartered or halved

- ¼ cup raspberries

- ¼ cup blueberries

- ½ apple, cored and cubed

- 1/4 small banana, sliced

- ½ plum, pitted and chopped

- ½ peach, pitted and chopped

- 1 tablespoon mint, chopped

- 1 mint flavored tea bag

- 1/2 tablespoon honey

- 1/4 tablespoon lemon juice

- 1/3 cup water

Instructions:

- Place 1/3 cup water in a small pan and bring to a boil. Add tea bag, honey and lemon juice.

- Simmer for 1 -2 minutes or until tea mixture reaches the strength you enjoy. Remove from the heat. Allow to cool. Mix all of the fruit together in a bowl. Pour the tea, honey and lemon juice mixture over the fruit. Mix together gently. Place fruit salad in the refrigerator to chill. Sprinkle the fresh mint over fruit salad before serving.

Honey Almond Peaches

Ingredients

- 1 can halved peaches, rinsed

- 2 tablespoons honey

- ½ cup low-fat ricotta cheese

- ¼ teaspoon cardamom

- ¼ cup almonds

Instructions:

- Rinse peach halves and arrange face up on baking sheet.

- Mix ricotta cheese thoroughly with honey and cardamom.

- Spoon honey-ricotta mixture into the peach halves.

- Bake peaches at 400 degrees for 15 minutes.

- Grind the almonds in a food processor until coarsely ground while the peaches are baking.

- Gently toast in a pan over medium heat.

Sprinkle with the course toasted almond meal after removing the peaches from the oven.

Pomegranate Poached Pears

Adapted from EatingWell

Makes: 4 servings

Active Time: 30 minutes

Total Time: 1 1/4 hours

Ingredients:

- 4 ripe, firm Bosc pears

- 1 1/2 cups pomegranate juice

- 1 cup sweet dessert wine, such as Muscatel or Riesling

- 1/2 cup pomegranate seeds, (1/2 large fruit)

- **Instructions:**

Peel pears, leaving them whole and stems intact. Slice off the bases so the pears will stand upright. Use an apple corer to remove cores, if desired, working from the base up.

Place the pears on their sides in a large saucepan or small Dutch oven. Pour pomegranate juice and wine over the pears. Bring to a simmer over medium-high heat. Cover, reduce heat to low and simmer gently until the pears are tender when pierced with the tip of a sharp knife, 30 to 45 minutes. Turn very gently once or twice as they cook so they color evenly. Using a slotted spoon, transfer the pears to a shallow bowl and set aside.

Boil the poaching liquid over high heat until the sauce is reduced to 1/2 cup, 15 to 20 minutes.

To serve, spoon 1 tablespoon sauce onto each of 4 dessert plates. Place a pear upright on each plate. Drizzle remaining sauce over each pear and sprinkle pomegranate seeds around it.

Tips & Notes

- Make Ahead Tip: Prepare through Step 3. Cover and refrigerate pears in sauce for up to 2 days. Serve at room temperature.

- Tip: Fill a large bowl with water. Hold the pomegranate in the water and slice off the crown. Lightly score the fruit into quarters, from crown to stem end. Keeping the fruit under water, break it apart, gently separating the plump seeds from the outer skin and white pith. The seeds will drop to the bottom of the bowl and the pith will float to the surface. Discard the pith. Pour the seeds into a colander. Rinse and pat dry.

Nutrition:

Per serving: 303 calories; 4 g fat (1 g sat, 2 g mono); 6 mg cholesterol; 53 g carbohydrates; 0 g added sugars; 2 g protein; 7 g fiber; 22 mg sodium; 559 mg potassium.

Greek Yogurt Cheesecake

adapted slightly from Eat Live Run

Ingredients:

Graham cracker crust (recipe below)

2 cups fat free plain Greek yogurt

1/2 cup sugar

pinch of salt

2 eggs

1 vanilla bean (seeds scraped out) or 2 tsp vanilla extract

1 T cornstarch

optional: sliced strawberries for garnish

Instructions:

Preheat oven to 350F. In a blender or food processor, combine the eggs, sugar, yogurt and vanilla. Blend until smooth, then add cornstarch and pinch of salt and blend again. Pour filling into crust in a 10 inch springform pan, and bake for 35 minutes.

When the cheesecake is done, it will still be jiggly in the center but will have a "done" look to it. The edges of the cake will start to pull away from the sides of the pan. Make sure you don't overbake.

Let cool then chill for 2-3 hours in the fridge before releasing springform.

Arrange the sliced strawberries over top of the cooled cheesecake and serve.

Simple Graham Cracker Crust

Around 1 1/2 cups graham cracker crumbs (about 10 sheets of graham crackers)

3 tablespoons almond milk. In a food processor, process crackers into fine crumbles. Add milk and process again to combine. Pour now-sticky crumbs into a prepared 10 inch springform pan, and smush down very firmly with your hands or a sheet of wax paper. You don't need to pre-bake the crust; just pour the filling straight in.

Italian Hazelnut Cookies

Makes: About 2 1/2 dozen cookies

Active Time: 15 minutes

Total Time: 2 hours

From Eating Well: These crispy cookies are made with Piedmontese staples—hazelnuts and eggs—and called Brutti Ma Buoni: literally, "Ugly But Good." But they are really more plain-looking than "ugly," and pack a powerful, sweet, nutty burst of flavor, making them welcome at any table.

Ingredients:

- 2 cups hazelnuts, toasted and skinned (see Tip)

- 1 1/4 cups sugar

- 4 large egg whites

- 1/2 teaspoon salt

- 1 teaspoon vanilla extract

Instructions:

- Position 2 racks as close to the center of the oven as possible; preheat to 325°F. Line 2 baking sheets with parchment paper or nonstick baking mats.

- Pulse nuts and sugar in a food processor until finely ground. Scrape into a large bowl.

- Beat egg whites and salt in another large bowl with an electric mixer on high speed until stiff peaks form. Using a rubber spatula, gently fold the egg whites into the nut mixture. Add vanilla and gently but thoroughly mix until combined.

- Drop the batter by the tablespoonful 2 inches apart on the prepared baking sheets.

- Bake the cookies until golden brown, switching the pans back to front and top to bottom halfway through, 25 to 30 minutes. Let cool on the baking sheets for 5 minutes. Gently transfer the cookies to a wire rack to cool completely. When the baking sheets are thoroughly cooled, repeat with the remaining batter.

Tips & Notes

- Make Ahead Tip: Store in an airtight container for up to 1 week. | Equipment: Parchment paper or nonstick baking mats

- Tip: Toast whole hazelnuts on a baking sheet in a 350°F oven, stirring occasionally, until fragrant, 7 to 9 minutes. Let the nuts cool for a few minutes, then rub together in a clean kitchen towel to remove most of the papery skins.

Nutrition:

Per cookie: 88 calories; 5 g fat (0 g sat, 4 g mono); 0 mg cholesterol; 10 g carbohydrates; 2 g protein; 1 g fiber; 46 mg sodium; 61 mg potassium.

Carbohydrate Servings: 1/2

Exchanges: 1 other carbohydrate, 1 fat

My name is Valerie Childs . . .

And I love people.

My purpose in life is to help as many people as possible reach their greatest potential physically, emotionally and spiritually.

As a life coach and nutrition coach, I've have for years coached in small groups and 1 on 1 until one day I realized this is not helping the multitudes of people I dreamed of helping.

I also found I was doing people a disservice by not putting down on paper all my years of knowledge and experience about what really works when it comes to weight loss, true natural health, and the importance of loving ourselves.

My heart breaks for people with destructive patterns that slowly kill them on the inside. Patterns such as terrible eating habits, (food) addictions, people whom never stop dieting, women and men who are never satisfied with the person they see in the mirror no matter how much they improve.

You know how they say many foods are terrible for us, the so-called "silent killers". The true silent killer however is really our own self. The feeling of never being good enough.

I want to make a change in the world. To provide true information about natural health, weight loss and overall well-being.

I know that by reading and applying the weight loss strategies I have provided you with in my books, you will lose weight. You will fit into your jeans and dresses again.

But more importantly, I hope by being acquainted with me you can finally start the journey of loving yourself. That when you look yourself in the mirror you will see how beautiful you are, no matter what size or what the number on the scale says.

My hope for you is that you will start SEEING yourself, the person you, how wonderfully made you are, and that you'll discover your unique purpose in life.

I talk about all of these important subjects in my newsletter, so make sure you're signed up to receive them. (You'll also get notified when I have books out for free).

xx Valerie

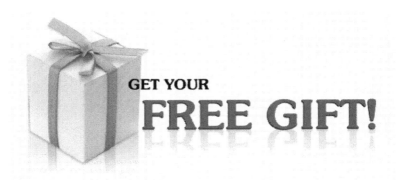

WAIT! – DO YOU LIKE FREE BOOKS?

My **FREE Gift** to You!! As a way to say **Thank You** for downloading my book, I'd like to offer you more **FREE BOOKS!** Each time we release a NEW book, we offer it first to a small number of people as a test–drive. Because of your commitment here in downloading my book, I'd love for you to be a part of this group. You can join easily here ➜ http://rapidslimdown.com/

Conclusion

Thank you again for downloading this book!

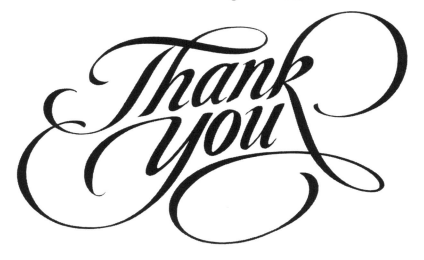

If you enjoyed this book, then I'd like to ask you for a favor, would you be kind enough to leave a review for this book on Amazon? It'd be greatly appreciated!

Help us better serve you by sending questions or comments to greatreadspublishing@gmail.com - Thank you!

Made in the USA
Lexington, KY
15 August 2015